Comparative Effectiveness Review

Number 130

Benefits and Harms of Routine Preoperative Testing: Comparative Effectiveness

Prepared for:
Agency for Healthcare Research and Quality
U.S. Department of Health and Human Services
540 Gaither Road
Rockville, MD 20850
www.ahrq.gov

Contract No. 290-2012-0012-I

Prepared by:
Brown Evidence-based Practice Center
Providence, RI

Investigators:
Ethan M. Balk, M.D., M.P.H.
Amy Earley, B.S.
Nira Hadar, M.S.
Nirav Shah, M.D.
Thomas A. Trikalinos, M.D., Ph.D.

AHRQ Publication No. 14-EHC009-EF
January 2014

This report is based on research conducted by the Brown Evidence-based Practice Center (EPC) under contract to the Agency for Healthcare Research and Quality (AHRQ), Rockville, MD (Contract No. 290-2012-0012-I). The findings and conclusions in this document are those of the authors, who are responsible for its contents; the findings and conclusions do not necessarily represent the views of AHRQ. Therefore, no statement in this report should be construed as an official position of AHRQ or of the U.S. Department of Health and Human Services.

The information in this report is intended to help health care decisionmakers—patients and clinicians, health system leaders, and policymakers, among others—make well informed decisions and thereby improve the quality of health care services. This report is not intended to be a substitute for the application of clinical judgment. Anyone who makes decisions concerning the provision of clinical care should consider this report in the same way as any medical reference and in conjunction with all other pertinent information, i.e., in the context of available resources and circumstances presented by individual patients.

This report may be used, in whole or in part, as the basis for development of clinical practice guidelines and other quality enhancement tools, or as a basis for reimbursement and coverage policies. AHRQ or U.S. Department of Health and Human Services endorsement of such derivative products may not be stated or implied.

This report may periodically be assessed for the urgency to update. If an assessment is done, the resulting surveillance report describing the methodology and findings will be found on the Effective Health Care Program Web site at: www.effectivehealthcare.ahrq.gov. Search on the title of the report.

This document is in the public domain and may be used and reprinted without permission. Citation of the source is appreciated.

Persons using assistive technology may not be able to fully access information in this report. For assistance contact EffectiveHealthCare@ahrq.hhs.gov.

Suggested citation: Balk EM, Earley A, Hadar N, Shah N, Trikalinos TA. Benefits and Harms of Routine Preoperative Testing: Comparative Effectiveness. Comparative Effectiveness Review No. 130. (Prepared by Brown Evidence-based Practice Center under Contract No. 290-2012-0012-I.) AHRQ Publication No. 14-EHC009-EF. Rockville, MD: Agency for Healthcare Research and Quality; January 2014. www.effectivehealthcare.ahrq.gov/reports/final.cfm.

Preface

The Agency for Healthcare Research and Quality (AHRQ), through its Evidence-based Practice Centers (EPCs), sponsors the development of systematic reviews to assist public- and private-sector organizations in their efforts to improve the quality of health care in the United States. These reviews provide comprehensive, science-based information on common, costly medical conditions, and new health care technologies and strategies.

Systematic reviews are the building blocks underlying evidence-based practice; they focus attention on the strength and limits of evidence from research studies about the effectiveness and safety of a clinical intervention. In the context of developing recommendations for practice, systematic reviews can help clarify whether assertions about the value of the intervention are based on strong evidence from clinical studies. For more information about AHRQ EPC systematic reviews, see www.effectivehealthcare.ahrq.gov/reference/purpose.cfm.

AHRQ expects that these systematic reviews will be helpful to health plans, providers, purchasers, government programs, and the health care system as a whole. Transparency and stakeholder input are essential to the Effective Health Care Program. Please visit the Web site (www.effectivehealthcare.ahrq.gov) to see draft research questions and reports or to join an email list to learn about new program products and opportunities for input.

We welcome comments on this systematic review. They may be sent by mail to the Task Order Officer named below at: Agency for Healthcare Research and Quality, 540 Gaither Road, Rockville, MD 20850, or by email to epc@ahrq.hhs.gov.

Richard G. Kronick, Ph.D.
Director, Agency for Healthcare Research
 and Quality

Jean Slutsky, P.A., M.S.P.H.
Director, Center for Outcomes and Evidence
Agency for Healthcare Research and Quality

Stephanie Chang, M.D., M.P.H.
Director, EPC Program
Center for Outcomes and Evidence
Agency for Healthcare Research and Quality

Elisabeth U. Kato, M.D., M.R.P.
Task Order Officer
Center for Outcomes and Evidence
Agency for Healthcare Research and Quality

Key Informants

In designing the study questions, the EPC consulted several Key Informants who represent the end-users of research. The EPC sought the Key Informant input on the priority areas for research and synthesis. Key Informants are not involved in the analysis of the evidence or the writing of the report. Therefore, in the end, study questions, design, methodological approaches, and/or conclusions do not necessarily represent the views of individual Key Informants.

Key Informants must disclose any financial conflicts of interest greater than $10,000 and any other relevant business or professional conflicts of interest. Because of their role as end-users, individuals with potential conflicts may be retained. The TOO and the EPC work to balance, manage, or mitigate any conflicts of interest.

The list of Key Informants who participated in developing this report follows:

Deepak L. Bhatt, M.D., M.P.H.
Department of Cardiology
VA Boston Healthcare System
Harvard Medical School
Boston University School of Medicine
Boston, MA

Steven R. Brown, M.D., FAAFP
American Academy of Family Physicians
University of Arizona College of Medicine
Phoenix, AZ

Nick Fitterman, M.D., FACP, SFHM
American College of Physicians
North Shore Long Island Jewish Health System
Westbury, NY

Barbara Gold, M.D., M.S.
American Society of Anesthesiology
University of Minnesota
Minneapolis, MN

Bernice Hecker, M.D., M.H.A., FACC
CMS Contractor Medical Director
Noridian Healthcare Solutions
Fargo, ND

Mark E. Mattingly, M.D., FCCP
Hospitalist Program
Medical Affairs, Blue Cross & Blue Shield of RI
Providence, RI

John B. Pollard, M.D.
Department of Anesthesia
VA Palo Alto Health Care System
Palo Alto, CA

Susan E. Pories, M.D., FACS
Department of Surgery
Mount Auburn Hospital
Harvard Medical School
Cambridge, MA

Pamela Wescott, M.P.P.
Patient Perspectives
Informed Medical Decisions Foundation
Boston, MA

Technical Expert Panel

In designing the study questions and methodology at the outset of this report, the EPC consulted several technical and content experts. Broad expertise and perspectives were sought. Divergent and conflicted opinions are common and perceived as healthy scientific discourse that results in a thoughtful, relevant systematic review. Therefore, in the end, study questions, design, methodologic approaches, and/or conclusions do not necessarily represent the views of individual technical and content experts.

Technical Experts must disclose any financial conflicts of interest greater than $10,000 and any other relevant business or professional conflicts of interest. Because of their unique clinical or content expertise, individuals with potential conflicts may be retained. The TOO and the EPC work to balance, manage, or mitigate any potential conflicts of interest identified.

The list of Technical Experts who participated in developing this report follows:

Steven R. Brown, M.D., FAAFP
American Academy of Family Physicians
University of Arizona College of Medicine
Phoenix, AZ

Nestor F. Esnaola, M.D., M.P.H., M.B.A., FACS
American Geriatrics Society, American College of Surgeons
Medical University of South Carolina
Charleston, SC

Nick Fitterman, M.D., FACP, SFHM
American College of Physicians
North Shore Long Island Jewish Health System
Westbury, NY

Lee A. Fleisher, M.D.
University of Pennsylvania Health System
Philadelphia, PA

Barbara Gold, M.D., M.S.
American Society of Anesthesiology
University of Minnesota
Minneapolis, MN

Bernice Hecker, M.D., M.H.A., FACC
CMS Contractor Medical Director
Noridian Healthcare Solutions
Fargo, ND

William Stuart Reynolds, M.D., M.P.H.
Department of Urologic Surgery
Female Pelvic Medicine and Reconstructive Surgery Center for Surgical Quality and Outcomes
Research
Vanderbilt University Medical Center
Nashville, TN

Pamela Thompson, M.S., MT(ASCP)
Division of Laboratory Science and Standards, American Society of Clinical Pathology
Centers for Disease Control and Prevention
Atlanta, GA

Peer Reviewers

Prior to publication of the final evidence report, EPCs sought input from independent Peer Reviewers without financial conflicts of interest. However, the conclusions and synthesis of the scientific literature presented in this report does not necessarily represent the views of individual reviewers.

Peer Reviewers must disclose any financial conflicts of interest greater than $10,000 and any other relevant business or professional conflicts of interest. Because of their unique clinical or content expertise, individuals with potential nonfinancial conflicts may be retained. The TOO and the EPC work to balance, manage, or mitigate any potential nonfinancial conflicts of interest identified.

The list of Peer Reviewers follows:

Rongwei (Rochelle) Fu, Ph.D.
Scientific Resource Center for the AHRQ Effective Health Care Program
Portland VA Research Foundation
Department of Public Health and Preventive Medicine
Oregon Health and Science University
Portland, OR

David I. Soybel, M.D.
Penn State Hershey Surgical Specialties
General Surgical & Surgical Oncology
Hershey, PA

Bobbie Jean Sweitzer, M.D.
Department of Anesthesia & Critical Care
University of Chicago
Chicago, IL

Benefits and Harms of Routine Preoperative Testing: Comparative Effectiveness

Structured Abstract

Objectives. Preoperative testing is used to guide the action plan for patients undergoing surgical and other procedures that require anesthesia and to predict potential postoperative complications. There is uncertainty whether routine or per-protocol testing in the absence of a specific indication prevents complications and improves outcomes, or whether it causes unnecessary delays, costs, and harms due to false-positive results.

Data sources. We searched MEDLINE® and Ovid Healthstar® (from inception to July 22, 2013), as well as Cochrane Central Trials Registry and Cochrane Database of Systematic Reviews.

Review methods. We included comparative and cohort studies of both adults and children undergoing surgical and other procedures requiring either anesthesia or sedation (excluding local anesthesia). We included all preoperative tests that were likely to be conducted routinely (in all patients) or on a per-protocol basis (in selected patients). For comparative studies, the comparator of interest was either no testing or ad hoc testing done at the discretion of the clinician. We also looked for studies that compared routine and per-protocol testing. The outcomes of interest were mortality, perioperative events, complications, patient satisfaction, resource utilization, and harms related to testing.

Results. Fifty-seven studies (14 comparative and 43 cohort) met inclusion criteria for the review. Well-conducted randomized controlled trials (RCTs) of cataract surgeries suggested that routine testing with electrocardiography, complete blood count, and/or a basic metabolic panel did not affect procedure cancellations (2 RCTs, relative risks [RRs] of 1.00 or 0.97), and there was no clinically important difference for total complications (3 RCTs, RR = 0.99; 95% confidence interval, 0.86 to 1.14). Two RCTs and six nonrandomized comparative studies of general elective surgeries in adults varied greatly in the surgeries and patients included, along with the routine or per-protocol tests used. They also mostly had high risk of bias due to lack of adjustment for patient and clinician factors, making their results unreliable. Therefore, they yielded insufficient evidence regarding the effect of routine or per-protocol testing on complications and other outcomes. There was also insufficient evidence for patients undergoing other procedures. No studies reported on quality of life, patient satisfaction, or harms related to testing.

Conclusions. There is high strength of evidence that, for patients scheduled for cataract surgery, routine preoperative testing has no effect on total perioperative complications or procedure cancellation. There is insufficient evidence for all other procedures and insufficient evidence comparing routine and per-protocol testing. There is no evidence regarding quality of life or satisfaction, resource utilization, or harms of testing and no evidence regarding other factors that may affect the balance of benefits and harms. The findings of the cataract surgery studies are not reliably applicable to other patients undergoing other higher risk procedures. Except arguably for cataract surgery, numerous future adequately powered RCTs or well-conducted and analyzed observational comparative studies are needed to evaluate the benefits and harms of routine preoperative testing in specific groups of patients with different risk factors for surgical and anesthetic complications undergoing specific types of procedures and types of anesthesia.

Contents

Tables

Figures

Appendixes

Executive Summary

Introduction

Traditionally, preoperative testing has been part of the preoperative care process to inform patient selection by determining fitness for anesthesia and identifying patients at high risk for perioperative complications. The American Society of Anesthesiologists (ASA) defines routine preoperative tests as those done in the absence of any specific clinical indication or purpose; they typically include a panel of blood tests, urine tests, chest radiography, and electrocardiogram (ECG).[1,2] These tests are performed to find latent abnormalities, such as anemia or silent heart disease, that could impact how, when, or whether the planned surgical procedure and concomitant anesthesia are performed. Many hospitals have instituted protocols to perform a series of laboratory tests prior to any operative procedure under the assumption that this information will enhance safety for surgical patients and reduce liability for adverse events.[2] During the past three decades, routine preoperative testing has been challenged by several academic publications with concerns about the sizable cost of testing, overtesting, the consequences of false-positive tests (leading to unnecessary workups and treatments), and the unknown benefit to patients.[3-8] In addition to increasing the cost of surgical care,[2] nonselective preoperative testing may result in false-positive or borderline results (in the absence of clinical indication), which require further investigation. Additional investigation may cause unnecessary psychological and economic burdens, postponement of surgery, and even morbidity and mortality (e.g., complications due to unnecessary biopsies performed to follow up false-positive laboratory tests).[2] As all routine testing does, preoperative testing will find some abnormal test results that will lead to new diagnoses (such as previously undetected lung cancer), but it is unclear whether the benefits accrued from responses to true-positive tests outweigh the harms of false-positive preoperative tests and, if there is a net benefit, how this benefit compares with the resource utilization required for testing.

Considerations for Evaluation of Preoperative Testing

Alternative Testing Strategies

There is no common terminology among anesthesiologists and surgeons regarding the alternative preoperative testing strategies. For this review, we define the three main alternatives as follows: (1) routine preoperative testing, in which the tests of interest are conducted in all patients undergoing a given procedure, regardless of medical history or other patient features; (2) per-protocol preoperative testing, in which the tests of interest are conducted in a subset of patients undergoing a given procedure, such as ECG only in patients aged ≥50 years or hemoglobin only in premenopausal women; (3) ad hoc, or elective, testing, in which preoperative testing is done at the discretion of the clinician doing a preoperative evaluation, based on patient history or physical examination (H&P) findings. No tests are done routinely or based on any protocol.

Preoperative Tests

There are many preoperative tests that can be ordered for a patient to determine fitness for surgery and anesthesia. Routine tests are those that may be of value to reduce the risk of procedural complications but are not directly related to the planned procedure. The specific tests under review here include hematologic, metabolic, and organ function blood tests; hemostasis tests; urinalysis; chest radiography (and related tests); ECG (and related tests); and pregnancy tests. These tests may be done alone (e.g., only a pregnancy test) or as part of a panel of tests.

Patient and Procedure Heterogeneity

Patients undergoing surgery show considerable variation in demographic characteristics, underlying health and comorbidities, indications for surgery, specific surgery planned, type of anesthesia planned (e.g., general vs. spinal anesthesia), and other factors. Differences among these factors may result in differences in the benefits of finding abnormalities (e.g., anemia) and in the potential harms of testing (e.g., delayed surgery or unnecessary colonoscopy). Therefore, it is important to look not only at the benefits and harms of preoperative testing in general, but also at specific patient and intervention (surgery-related) factors that might change the balance between the benefits and harms: namely, the risk of the surgical procedure, type of anesthesia planned, indication for surgery, comorbidities, and other patient characteristics.

The two most important factors are likely to be the risk of the procedure and the health status of the patient. The risk of procedural complications varies widely based on the type of surgery planned. It thus follows that the potential benefit of preoperative testing will vary based on the risk of complications related to the planned surgery. Although it has yet to be demonstrated, one could expect that some preoperative tests may be of greater value in predicting and ultimately reducing complications in higher rather than lower risk surgeries.

Similarly, one could expect that the risk of complications, and thus the potential value of preoperative testing, may be greater for patients with worse overall health status. The variation in the characteristics of patients undergoing surgery may lead to considerable differences in how abnormal preoperative test findings are handled, as well as their potential effect on surgery.

Clinician- and Setting-Based Differences

Inefficiencies in the preoperative testing processes or failures in the handoff of test results among primary care physicians, surgeons, and anesthesiologists ultimately affect the clinical utility of preoperative testing. Different hospitals, surgeons, and anesthesiologists have different protocols for obtaining preoperative testing, including, but not limited to, ad hoc testing by the surgeon or anesthesiologist, referral to the patient's primary care physician for testing at his or her discretion, and dedicated clinics with standardized protocols based on a patient's health status and planned surgery. Further, the comparator intervention, ad hoc testing, is by definition variable, depending on the clinician ordering the test, to what degree testing is based on any H&P he or she performs, and each clinician's likelihood of ordering few or many tests, which in part will be based on the local culture. Subsequent to testing, there is an implementation issue, in that any changes to patient outcomes due to testing must be mediated through clinical decisions about how to act on abnormal tests. Again, individual clinicians, different specialties, and different surgical settings are likely to have different thresholds for when and how to respond to abnormal tests. Examples include decisions about whether to delay or cancel surgery or whether to administer blood components preoperatively. This variability in care practices raises questions about whether ad hoc testing results in underutilization and/or overutilization of tests (balancing benefits and harms) compared with per-protocol testing, as well as whether testing ordered and followed up by different disciplines or types of clinicians has equivalent clinical utility.

Timing of Testing

A final factor that needs to be considered is the timing of the tests. Hospitals or surgical centers may dictate that preoperative testing must be done within a limited period before surgery, such as 30 days or 6 months. It is unknown whether there is adequate evidence to support any particular time threshold for preoperative tests.

Assessing Clinical Utility of Preoperative Testing

Preoperative testing can have a direct impact only on certain outcomes of interest, including emotional and cognitive changes in the patient conferred by testing and its results; any harms associated with the testing procedure (e.g., pain, hemorrhage, or bruising from a blood draw; exposure to ionizing radiation from imaging tests); and costs to the patient (in the form of time spent or copayments) or other types of resource utilization. For the most part, however, testing has indirect effects, including influencing treatment choices, delay or cancellation of the procedure (either appropriately to allow correction of or further treatment due to an abnormal test result or unnecessarily if no further treatment or evaluation was truly needed), and cascade testing (where abnormal tests lead to further appropriate or unnecessary tests).

Comparative studies of different preoperative testing strategies can effectively analyze all outcomes of interest. The range of outcomes that can be meaningfully assessed by noncomparative (cohort) studies, though, is more limited. Complication rates, the most important patient-centered outcome, can be adequately assessed only by comparative studies, since the underlying risk of complications will vary across cohorts of patients and types of surgery. The complication rate in a cohort study of routine testing is difficult to interpret in the absence of an estimate of the expected complication rate without routine testing. The only outcomes from cohort studies that can provide some information to address the Key Questions in this report are those directly related to the testing, such as surgery cancellation or delay due to an abnormal test result. However, this outcome is of somewhat limited value, since it does not address whether the patient benefited from or was harmed by the surgical cancellation or delay.

Statement of Work

Three professional medical associations nominated this topic for systematic review, citing the wide variation in clinical practice, the need for a guideline for routine preoperative testing, and the likelihood that a comparative effectiveness review on this subject would have broad clinical impact—particularly if such a review included the most commonly ordered tests in healthy patients, as well as those with comorbidities, undergoing a wide variety of high- and low-risk surgeries. The target audience for this review includes surgeons, anesthesiologists, and other clinicians involved in perioperative care of surgical patients; policymakers, including clinical practice guideline developers and surgical clinic administrators involved in determining preoperative testing policies and protocols; health care payers; researchers with an interest in perioperative care; and, ultimately, patients undergoing surgical procedures.

The review focuses on the direct evidence (evidence regarding actual changes in patient outcomes and management) of the comparative value of routine preoperative testing versus not testing (or other protocols for testing). This evidence is derived primarily from studies that directly compare testing protocols. These are the only studies that can demonstrate whether uniformly testing an unselected population prior to surgery leads to better outcomes for those patients. We also included cohort studies that report rates of "process outcomes" (rates of surgery cancellation, changes to planned surgery or anesthesia, etc.) only for patients being tested, since the rate of procedure delay, cancellation, and other changes due to testing is, by definition, zero in patients who do not undergo testing.

The review does not evaluate questions that, while important and related to the topic at hand, do not provide direct evidence of the comparative value of testing versus not testing. The review does not evaluate analyses that would require assumptions about what might have occurred without testing or assumptions about how testing might improve outcomes based on different rates of complications among patients with abnormal and normal preoperative tests. Specifically—

- We do not base assessments of the benefits and harms of preoperative testing on the incidence of perioperative complications (such as major bleeding) in studies that report only on patients who underwent testing (i.e., noncomparative studies). While these studies make conclusions regarding the possible value of testing, they do not provide evidence regarding the actual effect of routine preoperative tests, since the complication rates absent routine testing are unknown.
- We do not systematically review the prevalence rates of abnormal test results for different populations of patients undergoing surgery. These data do not provide evidence that ordering the test would alter perioperative outcomes, since the effect of acting on the abnormal test result on perioperative outcomes is unknown.
- We do not systematically review the test performance (e.g., sensitivity and specificity) of any of the tests because, again, the effect on perioperative outcomes of acting on the true or false abnormal test result is unknown.
- We do not assesses test results (i.e., abnormal vs. normal) as predictors of outcomes. The goal of this review is to assess whether actually ordering routine preoperative tests alters care and patient outcomes, and association studies do not provide data on how the test performs in different populations or the balance of benefits and harms.

Key Questions

We address the following Key Questions:

Key Question 1: How do routine or per-protocol preoperative testing strategies compare to no testing or alternative testing strategies with respect to outcomes—including perioperative clinical outcomes, quality of life or satisfaction, periprocedural patient management decisions, and resource utilization—among patients undergoing elective surgical procedures? How do outcomes vary by
   a. The risk of the surgical procedure, the type of anesthesia planned, the indication for surgery, comorbidities, or other patient characteristics?
   b. The structure of testing (e.g., routine for everyone vs. per protocol, whether testing is conducted in a specialized preoperative clinic) or who orders the tests (e.g., surgeon vs. anesthesiologist vs. primary care physician)?
   c. The length of time prior to the procedure that the tests are conducted?

Key Question 2: What are the harms of routine or per-protocol preoperative testing strategies compared to no testing or to alternative testing strategies? How do outcomes vary by:

a. The risk of the surgical procedure, the type of anesthesia planned, the indication for surgery, comorbidities, or other patient characteristics?
b. The structure of testing (e.g., routine for everyone vs. per protocol, whether testing is conducted in a specialized preoperative clinic) or who orders the tests (e.g., surgeon vs. anesthesiologist vs. primary care physician)?

Analytic Framework

To guide the development of the Key Questions for the evaluation of preoperative testing, we developed an analytic framework (Figure A) that maps the specific linkages associating the populations of interest, the interventions, the outcomes of interest (including harms), and the potential modifying factors. Specifically, this analytic framework depicts the chain of logic that the evidence must support to link the interventions to improved health outcomes.

Figure A. Analytic framework for routine preoperative testing

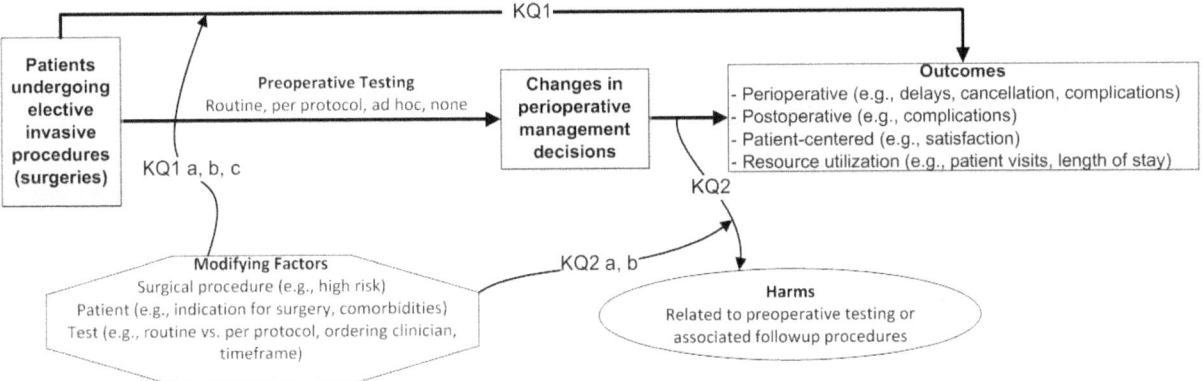

KQ = Key Question.

Methods

During a phase of topic refinement, in preparation for conducting this comparative effectiveness review, we convened a panel of Key Informants (including domain experts in anesthesia, general and breast surgery, and cardiology; health care payers with an interest in preoperative testing; a patient advocate; and representatives from the three topic nominators) and local domain experts (including an epidemiologist, internist, anesthesiologist, ophthalmologist, radiologist, and a thoracic and general surgeon). These individuals helped the team develop the Key Questions and the scope of work. We convened a Technical Expert Panel (TEP), which included experts in anesthesia, general surgery, urology, cardiology, internal medicine, and family medicine. The TEP provided input to help refine the protocol, identify important issues, and define parameters for the review of evidence. The TEP was also asked to suggest additional studies.

We conducted literature searches of studies in MEDLINE® and Ovid Healthstar® (from inception to July 22, 2013), as well as the Cochrane Central Trials Registry and Cochrane Database of Systematic Reviews (through the second quarter of 2013). The reference lists of prior systematic reviews and relevant guidelines were hand-searched. All citations were screened to identify articles relevant to each Key Question. The search included terms for surgical procedures, preoperative care, and diagnostic tests, including the specific tests ECG, chest radiography, blood counts, coagulation tests, biochemistry, glucose, urinalysis, kidney function tests, liver function tests, pregnancy tests, hemoglobinopathies, and pulmonary function tests.

Three team members double-screened all abstracts after an iterative training period to ensure that all screeners agreed upon the eligibility criteria. Full-text articles were retrieved for all potentially relevant articles. These were rescreened for eligibility. All rejected articles were confirmed by the team leader.

Population and Condition of Interest

We included studies conducted in both adults (≥18 years) and children undergoing surgical procedures requiring either anesthesia or sedation, including:

- Patients undergoing any elective or ambulatory surgical or other invasive procedure that commonly requires anesthesia or sedation of any type or approach that is administered by an anesthesia team member. Cataract surgery was included regardless of local practice regarding anesthesia or sedation.
- Procedures in any setting, including inpatient, outpatient, and office based.
- Any category of risk for surgical or anesthetic complications.
- Surgical procedures in any risk category, ranging from minor and minimally invasive through high-risk, maximally invasive surgeries (e.g., vascular, neurologic, thoracic, abdominal, and pelvic surgeries).

Patients undergoing nonsurgical diagnostic procedures that may require anesthesia or sedation (e.g., biopsy, colonoscopy) were excluded.

Interventions of Interest

We included all preoperative tests that we, our local expert, and the TEP agreed were likely to be conducted routinely or on a per-protocol basis. These included basic laboratory tests, simple radiography, and selected other relatively simple diagnostic tests.

The tests had to have been conducted in the preoperative period for the purpose of assessing the patient's risk and status prior to the planned procedure. We excluded tests performed for the purpose of diagnosis or staging of the disease for which the surgery was being performed or for specific surgical planning. We also excluded patient factors other than tests, including patient history, symptoms, physical examination signs or findings, and demographic features, or panels of "tests" that included any of these factors. While patient symptoms, such as decompensated congestive heart failure, may be important reasons for altering, delaying, or canceling surgery, they should be routinely assessed as part of an appropriate standard of care. In addition, for a given surgical procedure or set of procedures, the tests had to have been conducted either routinely (i.e., in all patients undergoing the procedure, regardless of age, sex, or medical condition) or based on a standard protocol (i.e., in all patients who met certain predetermined criteria based on age, sex, medical condition, or other factors).

Intervention and comparator arms were sorted into four categories: routine (everyone was scheduled to have all tests), per protocol (a protocol was used to determine who had which tests), ad hoc (testing was done at a clinician's discretion), or no testing. The distinction between routine and per-protocol testing was not always clear. If a study did not report sufficient information to distinguish the two, we assumed that routine testing was conducted. In a few instances, when a large number of tests were done routinely and a single test (e.g., ECG) was done per protocol, we also categorized this as routine testing.

Comparators of Interest

Comparators of interest included no preoperative testing (of a panel of tests or an individual test); ad hoc testing (i.e., the tests were conducted at the discretion of the ordering clinician, regardless of the reason); per-protocol testing (as a comparator to routine testing); a different panel of routine tests; testing conducted in a different setting or by a different type of clinician (e.g., in a specialized preoperative testing clinic vs. by the patient's primary care physician); and testing done at different presurgery time points (e.g., within 30 days vs. within 6 months).

Outcomes of Interest

For Key Question 1, outcomes were confined to those related to the conduct of the surgical procedures and anesthesia, perioperative events, patient satisfaction, and resource utilization. Specifically, they included clinical and other patient-centered outcomes (procedure or anesthesia delay, procedure cancellation, perioperative outcomes, including mortality and surgical complications); quality of life; satisfaction; patient resources; unplanned hospital readmission; change in disposition of care after surgery; length of hospital stay; other resource utilization, such as additional testing induced by a positive test or treatments for perioperative complications; and an intermediate outcome (changes to perioperative patient management other than procedure delay or cancellation). For Key Question 2, outcomes of interest included adverse events or harms related to testing, including complications of followup testing or treatment of abnormal test results, or poor outcomes related to delaying or canceling a procedure.

Eligible Study Designs

We included published peer-reviewed articles. We included studies that covered any timeframe, although they had to be longitudinal in design to the extent that testing was done prior to the planned procedure and followup occurred at least up to the time of the procedure.

We included comparative studies (in which one or more protocols for testing were compared with other protocols for testing, including protocols for no testing), whether randomized controlled trials (RCTs) or nonrandomized studies. We included both prospective and retrospective studies.

Because we expected the comparative studies to be limited in quantity and quality, we also evaluated cohort (noncomparative single-group) studies in which all study participants had the same testing battery or protocol. However, we limited these studies to those that reported "process" outcomes in which the process of care was altered, including procedure or anesthesia delay; procedure cancellation; and other resource utilization, such as unplanned followup tests or procedures and changes to perioperative patient management. As discussed above in the Statement of Work section, rates of other outcomes without a comparator would not provide interpretable data about the true benefits or harms of routine testing.

Data Extraction

Data from each study were extracted by one experienced methodologist. The extraction was reviewed and confirmed by at least one other methodologist. Data were extracted into customized forms in the Systematic Review Data Repository™ at srdr.ahrq.gov.

Quality Assessment

We assessed the methodological quality of studies based on predefined criteria. We used a three-category grading system (low, medium, or high risk of bias) to denote the methodological quality of each study. This system defines a generic grading scheme that is applicable to varying study designs, including RCTs, nonrandomized studies, and cohort studies.

Low risk of bias. These studies have the least apparent bias, and their results are considered valid. They generally possess the following: a clear description of the population, setting, interventions, and comparison groups; appropriate measurement of outcomes; appropriate statistical and analytic methods and reporting; no reporting errors; clear reporting of dropouts and a dropout rate less than 20 percent; and no obvious bias.

Medium risk of bias. These studies are susceptible to some bias, but it is not sufficient to invalidate the results. They do not meet all the criteria for low risk of bias due to some deficiencies, but none are likely to introduce major bias. They may be missing information, making it difficult to assess limitations, including risk of bias per se, and potential problems.

High risk of bias. These studies have been judged to carry a significant risk of bias that may invalidate the reported findings. These studies have serious errors in design, analysis, or reporting and contain discrepancies in reporting or have large amounts of missing information.

Minimal Important Difference

With input from the TEP, we made a priori definitions of minimal important differences (MIDs). The MID is a clearly defined clinical threshold, below which the evidence (effect estimates and corresponding confidence intervals [CIs]) shows no meaningful difference and above which the evidence shows a benefit or harm of one intervention over another. For mortality and major or severe life- or health-altering morbidities and complications (such as stroke, myocardial infarction, or life-threatening hemorrhage), the MID is 0 percent because any difference is of concern to patients and clinicians for this low-risk (generally low-cost) intervention (preoperative testing). However, to make the determination that there is evidence of no difference, we used a threshold of 20 percent on the relative risk (RR) scale. For other, noncritical outcomes, we also used an MID of 20 percent, based on agreement that smaller differences would not be clinically important.

Grading the Body of Evidence

We graded the strength of the body of evidence, in accordance with the AHRQ "Methods Guide for Effectiveness and Comparative Effectiveness Reviews,"[9] based on risk of bias, consistency across studies, directness of the evidence, precision (based on the MID), and risk of reporting bias. The strength of evidence was ranked as either high, moderate, low, or insufficient. Ratings were assigned based on our level of confidence that the evidence reflected the true effect for the major comparisons of interest. We further assessed the body of evidence regarding its applicability to the U.S. population of patients undergoing surgical procedures.

Results

The literature search yielded 4,581 citations. From these, 220 articles were provisionally accepted for review based on abstracts and titles. After screening the full text, 57 studies (in 58 articles) were found to have met the inclusion criteria. Fourteen of the 57 were comparative, and the remainder were single-group studies. Three RCTs focused on cataract surgery, two RCTs and six nonrandomized studies focused on general or various surgeries, one RCT focused on vascular surgery, and one nonrandomized study each focused on tonsillectomy and orthopedics. Overall, the studies evaluated the preoperative tests for the following procedures: general or various surgeries (37 studies), tonsillectomy (5 studies), cataract surgery (4 studies), orthopedic surgery (4 studies), vascular surgery (3 studies), head and neck/ear, nose, throat surgery (2 studies), and 1 study each for neurosurgery and electroconvulsive therapy. Seventeen of the studies were conducted in children, 25 in adults, and 15 in a mixed population of adults and children. Forty studies were published before 2000, including 7 of the 14 comparative studies; 17 studies were published after 2000. Thirteen studies had a high risk of bias, 10 had a medium risk of bias, and 34 had a low risk of bias.

The preoperative tests evaluated in the studies fall into the following categories: basic metabolic panel (electrolytes, kidney function, glucose); extended metabolic panel (liver function tests and other serum tests); blood counts (including hemoglobin, hematocrit, white blood cells, and platelets); hemostasis tests (including prothrombin time, partial thromboplastin time, and bleeding time); urinalysis; pregnancy tests; ECG; chest x ray (CXR); pulmonary function testing; and echocardiography.

Comparative Studies

Cataract Surgery

Three RCTs—two with low, one with moderate risk of bias—compared routine versus no (or ad hoc) preoperative testing with ECG, basic metabolic panel, and complete blood count (CBC) for patients undergoing cataract surgery. The studies were clinically similar to each other and consistent; there is a high strength of evidence of no clinically important difference in complication rates. By meta-analysis, for total complications, the RR is 0.99 (95% CI, 0.86 to 1.14). There is also a high strength of evidence suggesting that routine testing does not affect rates of procedure cancellation, but the confidence intervals were too wide to definitely exclude a clinically important difference: RR=1.00 (95% CI, 0.42 to 2.38) and 0.97 (95% CI, 0.78 to 1.21). No other outcomes were reported. The evidence is inadequate to evaluate potential differences based on subgroups of patients. Overall, there is no evidence of different outcomes related to routine preoperative testing.

General or Various Surgeries, Adults

One RCT with low risk of bias and four nonrandomized studies with high risk of bias compared routine testing (two studies) or per-protocol testing (three studies) with ad hoc testing, using ECG, CXR, basic and extended metabolic panels, CBC, hemostasis tests, and urinalysis in adult patients undergoing a broad range of elective surgeries. A sixth study compared time periods when patients were to receive either routine testing, during a retrospective period, or per-protocol testing, during a prospective period, with a large number of tests. None of the nonrandomized studies adjusted for baseline differences in patient characteristics, types of surgery, surgeons or anesthesiologists, their experience, or other confounders. They also did not analyze how or whether the routine or per-protocol tests were linked to resulting outcomes (complications). The RCT reported only on complications, of which there were only a small number; therefore, this trial was underpowered to provide any reliable estimate of relative differences in complications. We have no confidence in the estimate of effects across these studies due to these methodological deficiencies, the important clinical heterogeneity (differences) across all studies, and the high risk of bias of the nonrandomized studies (particularly related to lack of necessary adjustments). Therefore, there is insufficient evidence regarding perioperative complications. There is also insufficient evidence of a clinically significant difference in the rate of perioperative death. The clinical heterogeneity of studies, without reporting of subgroup analyses of patients or procedures within studies, further precludes a conclusion about which patients would benefit from routine testing. There is also insufficient evidence regarding other specific outcomes, including return to the operating room, prolonged hospital stay, or surgical cancellation or delay. No trial reported on quality of life or satisfaction, change in anesthesia or procedure plan, or resource utilization. A single nonrandomized study with high risk of bias provided insufficient evidence regarding the comparison of routine and per-protocol testing. Given the deficiencies in the evidence across studies, it was not possible to compare the effects of routine and per-protocol testing. No trial addressed Key Question 2 regarding harms of routine preoperative testing. The evidence is inadequate to evaluate potential differences based on subgroups of interest.

Orthopedic Surgery, Adults

There is insufficient evidence regarding the comparison of routine versus per-protocol preoperative testing in adults undergoing orthopedic surgery. A single retrospective nonrandomized study with high risk of bias found no difference in the rate of unplanned hospital admissions within 30 days of surgery.

Vascular Surgery, Adults

There is insufficient evidence regarding the comparison of routine versus per-protocol preoperative testing in adults undergoing vascular surgery. A single RCT with low risk of bias failed to find differences in rates of perioperative death or cardiac complications.

General or Various Surgeries, Children

One RCT from 1975 with medium risk of bias reported limited outcome data. A retrospective nonrandomized study with high risk of bias failed to provide sufficient evidence regarding the effect on patient and resource outcomes of routine or per-protocol preoperative testing. The limited data suggest no difference in length of hospital stay related to routine testing with basic and extended metabolic panels and a counterintuitive increase in minor perioperative complications with routine preoperative testing. The age of the studies (38 and 15 years) further calls into question the applicability of their findings to modern pediatric surgical management. No study reported on quality of life, satisfaction, surgical delay, change in anesthesia or procedure plan, resource utilization, or harms of routine testing. The evidence is inadequate to evaluate potential differences based on subgroups of interest.

Tonsillectomy and/or Adenoidectomy, Children

There is insufficient evidence regarding routine or per-protocol preoperative testing in children undergoing tonsillectomy and/or adenoidectomy. A single flawed retrospective nonrandomized study that is 16 years old found significantly higher rates of perioperative bleeding among patients of less experienced surgeons who routinely conducted hemostasis tests than those of more experienced surgeons who performed per-protocol testing. However, none of the bleeding episodes were related to clinically significant abnormal coagulation tests, and the difference in bleeding rates was more likely to have been related to the experience and surgical volume of the surgeons.

Cohort Studies

Given how few comparative studies were available, we looked at cohort studies to test the indirect link between testing and outcomes, since if tests can be shown not to affect management, they cannot affect outcomes. The weaknesses with this approach are that it is not possible to determine if the change in management led to better or worse outcomes and that the implicit comparison can be made only with no testing. No implicit comparison can be made with ad hoc testing based on H&P, since there are no data on management changes based on the ad hoc testing. For the purposes of this section, we combined data from the true cohort studies and the routine or per-protocol arms from the comparative studies. This section focuses on the rates of specific outcomes, and the data from the comparative studies are equivalent to those from the cohort studies. Among the 57 studies eligible for this review, the 47 with relevant outcomes are summarized in this section.

The 47 studies report a total of five "process" outcomes of interest: change in patient management (4 studies conducted in adults); change in surgical technique (3 studies conducted in adults, 1 study conducted in children); change in anesthetic management (10 studies conducted in adults, 6 studies conducted in children); procedure cancellation (19 studies conducted in adults, 11 studies conducted in children); and procedure or anesthetic delay (19 studies conducted in adults, 7 studies conducted in children). Thirty-three (70%) of the studies were published before 2000. Except for a 5.1-percent rate of procedure delays in one study from 2005, all patient management changes that occurred in 2 percent or more of patients were in older studies. Thirty-nine (83%) of the studies evaluated routine preoperative testing; the other eight evaluated per-protocol testing. An important caveat for the analysis of these studies is that, in general, it is only implied that procedure changes or cancellations were truly due to abnormal test results as opposed to changes that may have occurred for reasons separate from testing. While this caveat also applies to the comparative studies, in these analyses there is no reference group for comparison.

With these caveats, the following conclusions can be made from the cohort studies. In all preoperative testing scenarios for which more than a single study was available (i.e., approaching a sufficient evidence base to form a conclusion), testing resulted in some changes in management. In other words, the evidence suggests that in most situations, routine preoperative testing will result in some delay or cancellation of the procedure (in most studies, <2%) or some changes to anesthetic management (up to 11%) or surgical procedure (<1%). However, it is not possible to say whether the changes led to benefit or harm for patients because, without a comparator group, one cannot assess how the changes in management may have been associated with perioperative outcomes. Two studies suggest that change in management from CXR is more common for older patients (primarily >60 years). Two other studies looked at CXR and ECG by sex and other factors. One of these studies suggests that the effect of ECG is similar in men and women, but the second study suggests that CXR results in change in management in more men, those in a higher ASA risk category, those with respiratory disease, and those with "major" surgeries planned (as opposed to "minor" or "standard" surgeries), particularly in patients undergoing thoracic, cardiac, and vascular surgeries. The studies were too clinically heterogeneous to ascertain whether there were any patterns suggesting a difference in process outcomes based on whether preoperative testing was conducted routinely or per protocol.

Discussion

Key Findings and Strength of Evidence

We identified 57 studies that reported clinically pertinent outcomes in patients who had routine or per-protocol preoperative testing performed. However, only 14 of the studies provided direct comparisons between routine or per-protocol testing and ad hoc or no testing, and only two studies compared routine with per-protocol testing. Furthermore, only seven of the comparative studies were RCTs, three of which were conducted in patients undergoing cataract surgery. The large majority of data come from cohort studies that provided evidence only about how frequently procedures or anesthesia were canceled, delayed, or altered in response to preoperative testing.

In summary, there is a high strength of evidence from three well-conducted RCTs that consistently found that, for patients scheduled for cataract surgery, preoperative ECG, metabolic panel (or glucose), and CBC have no effect on total perioperative complications or procedure cancellation (Table A). In contrast, there is insufficient evidence for the effect of routine preoperative testing in all other surgeries and populations. There is also insufficient evidence to estimate a difference in outcomes based on whether preoperative testing was conducted routinely or per protocol. There are one RCT and five nonrandomized studies of routine or per-protocol testing in adults undergoing various elective surgeries; however, the studies were highly heterogeneous in populations, elective surgeries, and tests used. Furthermore, the nonrandomized studies were all fundamentally flawed in that they failed to adjust for differences among study groups in the patients, surgeries, surgeons, anesthetics used, anesthesiologists, or other possible confounders. These studies generally found lower rates of postoperative complications and deaths among patients undergoing routine or per-protocol testing, but the heterogeneity and flaws in the studies preclude any confidence in the accuracy or validity of the findings. However, while there is no evidence regarding minimally invasive surgeries similar to cataract surgery, it may be valid to conclude that routine preoperative testing in these other low-risk surgeries would also have no effect.

There is insufficient evidence for all other categories of procedures and patients, for all other outcomes of interest, and regarding more detailed analyses of differences in how testing is performed. In particular, there is no comparative evidence regarding quality of life or satisfaction, resource utilization, or harms. Among comparative studies, there is insufficient reported evidence regarding how outcomes may differ in different subgroups of patients, or how the effect of preoperative testing may vary based on the risk of the surgical procedure or other factors.

The apparent difference in the effect of routine or per-protocol testing in patients undergoing cataract and general elective surgery is arguably not surprising. Cataract surgery is a very low-risk procedure, safe enough to be done in an ophthalmologist's office, that is minimally invasive and usually requires only local anesthesia with sedation. Other than increases in vagal tone, there is little reason to expect cardiac strain in the typical patient undergoing cataract surgery. While the patients are typically elderly, and thus have a relatively high rate of comorbidities, they are generally not suffering from any acute illnesses. In contrast, general elective surgeries in adults encompass a wide range of patients and surgeries, including many with acute or serious medical conditions requiring surgery and highly invasive cardiothoracic, abdominal, and vascular surgeries. These patients are intrinsically at higher risk of perioperative complications and thus, conceptually, may benefit most from preoperative tests that pick up correctable abnormalities that may be associated with complications.

Most of the evidence was from cohort studies. However, the nature of the intervention under consideration (preoperative testing) makes the lack of a direct comparator (ad hoc testing) among these studies particularly problematic in terms of interpreting the findings. Regardless of the specific preoperative tests used or how they are implemented, the rate of perioperative complications due to either the procedure or the anesthesia will always depend primarily on the underlying risks of the surgical procedure, the type of anesthesia used, the skill and experience of the surgeons and anesthesiologists, the medical condition of the patients, and the quality of perioperative care. The risk of perioperative complications when preoperative testing was conducted, without information about the risk of complications without testing (or only ad hoc testing), does not provide information on the effect of the testing on those risks. An adequate comparator that controls for the myriad factors that also impact perioperative complications is needed.

Study Limitations

Across nonrandomized studies, there was a lack of adjustment for possible confounders. All of the nonrandomized studies failed to control for cluster effects, particularly those related to individual surgeons or surgical experience. Six nonrandomized studies compared different time periods within an institution before or after implementation or removal of a preoperative testing policy. However, institutional differences between the time periods (such as incremental improvements in surgical techniques, anesthesia, or nursing care) were not accounted for. The bias that can result from the lack of adjustment (e.g., by propensity score) was best exemplified in the nonrandomized study that compared concurrent surgeries. In one of the two comparative studies comparing routine versus per-protocol testing with hemostasis tests on children undergoing tonsillectomy and/or adenoidectomy, the comparison was really between the bleeding complication rates of the 2 most experienced surgeons (who used a testing protocol in 2,624 children) and those of the 11 less experienced surgeons (who did routine testing in 1,750 children total). Arguably, the finding that perioperative bleeding was more common in the latter group provides evidence that surgical experience and skill are predictors of complications and says little or nothing about whether preoperative testing may (or may not) have prevented any bleeding episodes.

Intrinsic Limitations of Research on Preoperative Testing

Another limitation of the evidence that would be difficult to overcome also relates to the nature of the intervention. Preoperative testing does not in and of itself affect the outcomes of interest (except resource utilization and possibly quality of life/satisfaction, although there are no data on these outcomes). Instead, the preoperative tests potentially cause the health care providers to alter a patient's management—by implementing an intervention to correct or account for the abnormal test; by delaying, canceling, or changing the procedure or anesthesia; or by making changes to postoperative care. Additionally, the preoperative test may be useful for perioperative management to use as a reference (e.g., to know whether a measure has changed in a postoperative test compared with the preoperative test—for example, whether an ECG abnormality is new or not). Thus, the value of any preoperative test is fully dependent on the health care providers and their responses to abnormal tests. One could expect responses to vary among surgeons, anesthesiologists, primary care physicians, nurse practitioners, and other providers. One could also expect them to vary among individual providers across hospitals, settings (e.g., urban vs. rural), geographic regions, and a myriad of other health care provider variables. However, none of these factors were accounted for in the studies. This limitation further hampers the interpretation of the evidence, particularly from the cohort studies, but also arguably from the unadjusted nonrandomized studies.

Interpretation of the evidence is further complicated by the wide variability in clinical practice in the thoroughness of preoperative H&P (and whether it is done) and the general lack of reporting regarding H&P in the studies. This could have an important impact on what tests are conducted ad hoc (i.e., in the comparator arms of the studies). Rather than leading to more or less testing, it can lead to more appropriate testing, since the tendency to order tests based on a "shotgun" approach will be reduced. But H&P could be considered equivalent to a "test" performed by the clinician (instead of the laboratory or radiology technician), which may or may not have value independent of true preoperative tests. Furthermore, H&P is intrinsically nonstandardized and heterogeneous, depending on the specific questions asked and the details of the examination. Traditionally, H&Ps have been completed in the surgical clinics and on the day of surgery by the anesthesiology teams. More recently, preoperative assessment clinics staffed by perioperative medicine specialists are becoming more common. These clinics focus on optimizing patients for their perioperative course, and a thorough H&P is the cornerstone of that process. However, none of the studies specifically investigated testing in this setting.

Any management changes due to abnormal test results (and presumably any subsequent changes in perioperative outcomes) would logically be the same regardless of whether testing was done routinely, per protocol, or at the clinician's discretion. Therefore, the variability in ad hoc testing could have an important impact on the comparison of outcomes between ad hoc and routine or per-protocol testing. Without good descriptions in studies of typical H&P or the triggers to order ad hoc tests, it is difficult to interpret the applicability of the studies to the general (or any specific) population and the comparison among different testing regimens.

Limitations of Cohort Studies

Because of the underlying lack of interpretability of the complication rates in these studies, we restricted analyses to "process" outcomes related to decisions about whether the procedure or anesthesia was altered based on testing. These included cancellation or delay of surgery, changes in either the planned surgery or anesthesia, and overall changes in patient management. To the extent possible, based on the reported data, we focused on decisions that were made specifically because of test results (presumably abnormal results), but most studies did not clearly define their outcomes, requiring us to assume this was the case. However, the information to be gleaned from most of these studies was limited. When no procedures were canceled or delayed and no changes were made to either the planned procedure or anesthesia, it may be reasonable to conclude that the testing was of no value, at least up to the time that the procedure was performed. However, the assumption that the testing was of no value overall requires that the postoperative course also be unaffected by the availability of the preoperative tests. In reality, it is likely that some abnormal preoperative tests, such as an elevated glucose, would alter perioperative management, such as more intensive glucose monitoring.

Interpreting the finding that a certain (nonzero) percentage of procedures were canceled, delayed, or changed is not straightforward. First, one must make a conclusion as to whether the cancellations, delays, or changes were warranted. Second, one must make assumptions about whether the patients' outcomes were changed. If a procedure was canceled or delayed, at a certain level the patient's immediate health care was worsened, assuming the planned surgery was necessary. However, it is unknowable whether the delay or cancellation may have prevented a complication that would have been worse than the prolongation of the disease state necessitating surgery. Third, one must make a determination as to whether the testing led to changes in care sufficiently rarely (below some percentage threshold) that the testing is of sufficiently limited value to safely forgo it, or whether the changes in care occur frequently enough that they can be assumed to be an important tool or predictor regarding surgical management.

With these caveats, the following conclusions can be made from the cohort studies. In all cases where there are at least two studies (i.e., approaching a sufficient evidence base to form a conclusion), there was no test or set of tests used routinely for a similar population (adults or children) prior to a similar set of procedures for which the testing consistently resulted in no changes in management. In other words, the evidence suggests that in most situations, routine preoperative testing will result in some delay or cancellation of the procedure or some change to anesthetic management or surgical procedure. Again, whether these changes benefit or harm patients is unknown from these data. That said, the only studies that directly compared outcomes in subsets of patients were cohort studies that evaluated changes in patient management, including specialty consultations or nonsurgery-related changes in patient care. Two studies suggest that change in management from CXR is more common for older patients (primarily >60 years). Two other studies also looked at CXR and ECG by sex and other factors. One of these studies suggests that the effect of ECG is similar in men and women, but the second study suggests that CXR results in change in management in more men, those in a higher ASA risk category, those with respiratory disease, and those with "major" surgeries planned (as opposed to "minor" or "standard" surgeries), particularly in patients undergoing thoracic, cardiac, and vascular surgeries. However, given the small number of studies that compared outcomes in different subgroups of patients, together with the unknown connection between changing patient management and true patient outcomes, it is premature to conclude that the differences found are clinically important.

Table A. Routine or per-protocol preoperative testing: Findings and strength of evidence

Outcome	Surgery	Tests	Study Design (Risk of Bias)	Finding	Strength of Evidence
Perioperative complications, total	Cataract surgery	ECG, metabolic panel, CBC	RCT (2 low, 1 medium)	No effect of testing (summary RR = 0.99; 95% CI, 0.86 to 1.14).	High
	Various, adults (comparison: routine vs. ad hoc testing)	Multiple	RCT (1 low) NRS (4 high)	In most studies, fewer complications occurred with testing, but studies were highly heterogeneous and underpowered; not a clinically important difference.	Insufficient
	Various, adults (comparison: routine vs. per-protocol testing)	Multiple	NRS (1 high)	No events in either group.	Insufficient
	Various, children	Multiple†	NRS (1 high)	More complications occurred with testing, but not a clinically important difference.	Insufficient
	Vascular, adults	Stress echo	RCT (1 high)	No significant difference in cardiac events.	Insufficient
Perioperative death	Various, adults (comparison: routine vs. ad hoc testing)	Multiple	NRS (4 high)	In most studies, fewer deaths occurred with testing, but studies were highly heterogeneous and underpowered.	Insufficient
	Various, adults (comparison: routine vs. per-protocol testing)	Multiple	NRS (1 high)	No events in either group.	Insufficient
	Vascular, adults	Stress echo	RCT (1 high)	Cardiac and respiratory deaths were rare; no difference between groups.	Insufficient

Table A. Routine or per-protocol preoperative testing: Findings and strength of evidence (continued)

Outcome	Surgery	Tests	Study Design (Risk of Bias)	Finding	Strength of Evidence
Perioperative complications, major (total)	Various, children	Multiple†	NRS (1 high)	Imprecise estimate failing to support a difference.	Insufficient
Perioperative complications, specific (selected)	Various, adults (comparison: routine vs. ad hoc testing)	Multiple*	RCT (1 low) NRS (3 high)	Clinically important difference: fewer episodes of renal failure with testing (0.9% vs. 0%; 1 study). Significant but not clinically important difference: fewer episodes of pneumonia with testing (1 study). No significant differences for other complications, including any outcome from RCT.	Insufficient
	Various, adults (comparison: routine vs. per-protocol testing)	Multiple*	NRS (1 high)	No difference between groups, but only rare events.	Insufficient
	Various, children	Multiple†	NRS (1 high)	Clinically important difference: more episodes of persistent vomiting with testing (RR = 1.76; 95% CI, 1.22 to 2.54). Clinically important difference: more episodes of restlessness with testing (RR = 3.91; 95% CI, 2.19 to 6.97). No significant differences were found for other complications.	Insufficient
	Tonsillectomy, children (comparison: routine vs. ad hoc testing)	Coagulation tests	NRS (1 high)	No significant difference in bleeding complications.	Insufficient
Return to operating room	Various, adults	Multiple*	NRS (1 high)	No significant difference in rate of return to operating room.	Insufficient
Unplanned hospital admission	Orthopedic, adults	Multiple*	NRS (1 high)	No significant difference in rate of unplanned hospital admissions.	Insufficient
Procedure cancellation	Cataract surgery	ECG, metabolic panel, CBC	RCT (1 low, 1 medium)	Likely no effect of testing† (summary RR = 0.97; 95% CI, 0.79 to 1.20).	High

Table A. Routine or per-protocol preoperative testing: Findings and strength of evidence (continued)

Outcome	Surgery	Tests	Study Design (Risk of Bias)	Finding	Strength of Evidence
	Various, adults	Multiple*	NRS (1 high)	Possibly no effect of testing (RR = 0.93; 95% CI, 0.76 to 1.14).	Insufficient
	Various, children	Multiple†	NRS (1 high)	No effect of testing (no surgeries canceled).	Insufficient
Procedure delay	Various, adults	Multiple*	NRS (1 high)	No significant difference in procedure delay.	Insufficient
Length of stay	Various, adults	Multiple*	NRS (1 high)	No significant difference in length of stay.	Insufficient
	Various, children	Multiple†	RCT (1 medium) NRS (1 high)	No significant difference in length of stay.	Insufficient
Quality of life/satisfaction, anesthesia change, surgery change, resource utilization, or harms	None	Not applicable	No studies	None	Insufficient
Subgroup analyses	None	Not applicable	No studies	None	Insufficient

CBC = complete blood count, CI = confidence interval, ECG = electrocardiogram, NRS = nonrandomized comparative study, RCT = randomized controlled trial, RR = relative risk, Stress echo = dobutamine stress echocardiogram.

*ECG, chest x ray, basic and extended metabolic panels, CBC, coagulation tests, and urinalysis.

†Hemoglobin, urinalysis, creatine phosphokinase, and cholinesterase.

‡Just fails to meet 20% minimal important difference threshold for evidence of no difference.

Limitations of Systematic Review

We relied mainly on electronic database searches and perusal of reference lists to identify relevant studies. Unpublished relevant studies may have been missed. We also kept the review focused on the evidence that most directly addresses the comparative effect of routine or per-protocol preoperative testing versus ad hoc or no testing. Thus, we did not review the wide range of indirect evidence from which conclusions about whether testing might be of value might be inferred. The Statement of Work section in the Introduction spells out the broader research questions that were not addressed here. The decision to narrow the scope of the review was made in part due to time and resource constraints. Future updates of this review may be able to broaden the scope of the research questions, particularly if it remains the case that there are few eligible comparative studies.

The conclusions, to a large extent, reflect the limitations of the underlying evidence base. Our ability to address most of the issues raised by the Key Questions was hampered by a paucity or complete lack of data, particularly from comparative studies.

Applicability

In general, the applicability of the evidence is limited, with the exception of the studies of cataract surgery. The cataract RCTs all had similar findings, despite being conducted in different settings, in different countries, and with somewhat different eligibility criteria and study designs. Furthermore, the first trial was conducted in nearly 20,000 patients. This implies that the conclusion that there is no effect of routine testing with ECG, a basic metabolic panel, and blood counts for cataract surgery is likely to be broadly applicable. The applicability of the findings for adults undergoing a range of elective surgeries is less clear. The studies evaluated different tests in different populations receiving different surgical procedures and did not adequately report the conditions under which ad hoc testing was done (i.e., the extent of H&P or the triggers to order testing).

Evidence Gaps and Future Research

Table B summarizes the evidence gaps with regard to the two Key Questions and subquestions of this systematic review.

Table B. Evidence gaps

Key Question	Category	Evidence Gap
Beneficial effects of routine or per-protocol preoperative testing	General	For all procedures and surgeries requiring more than local anesthesia except cataract surgery, there is a paucity or lack of comparative studies to assess the value of the intervention.
	Population	Evidence is needed to evaluate the effect of testing for— All elective procedures except cataract surgery Specific procedures Different types of anesthesia Different aged populations—children, adults, and older adults Different preoperative health status, including comorbidities Different categories of anesthesia risk Existing studies generally provide poor descriptions of the patient populations—specific procedures planned, disease conditions, comorbidities, surgical and anesthesia risk categories, race, and other factors.
	Interventions and comparators	Difference in effect of routine testing (in all patients) vs. per-protocol testing (in selected patients). Effect of individual tests (within panels of tests) compared with effect of other individual tests. Different effects based on who ordered the test or the structure of testing (e.g., if done through a preanesthesia clinic or internist's office). These data are generally not reported. How long prior to the planned procedure tests can be performed (e.g., within 1 week or 6-12 months) and still provide a benefit (assuming the preoperative testing is beneficial).
	Outcomes	Major perioperative complications (to some degree in contrast with total complications). Quality of life or satisfaction. Resource utilization. Postoperative management. Perioperative complications: improved standardization is needed regarding which perioperative complications should be reported; however, the list of complications will vary depending on the procedure.
Harms of routine or per-protocol preoperative testing	General/outcomes	There is no evidence regarding harms of testing.
Subgroup analyses	General	No comparative studies provided subgroup analyses based on any baseline patient characteristics, procedures, anesthesia type, or other factors listed above under Population or Interventions and comparators.

For all procedures and surgeries requiring more than local anesthesia except cataract surgery, there is a paucity or lack of comparative studies to assess the value of the intervention. Evidence is needed to evaluate specific procedures and types of anesthesia, and specific populations, including patients at different surgical risk. Evidence is needed to compare routine testing versus per-protocol testing, the effect of individual tests, who orders and manages tests, and the timing of tests. Evidence is needed for all clinical outcomes, but it is particularly lacking for quality of life and satisfaction, resource utilization, and harms.

A large series of RCTs would best address the important research questions regarding routine and per-protocol preoperative testing. Focused studies evaluating specific tests or panels of tests in well-defined patients undergoing a narrow set of procedures will be of greater value to clinicians and decisionmakers deciding who should be routinely tested preoperatively than less focused studies. Conducting a series of such trials appears to be quite feasible, given the large number of elective procedures performed at many hospitals or surgical clinics; the low cost of the intervention (since in many situations the trial will primarily involve randomizing patients to either receive tests that are already available to them or to withhold those tests, as opposed to requiring resources to cover the costs of additional interventions); and the short term of the postoperative followup that is required (during hospitalization or up to 1 to 3 months). Trials should collect sufficient data to effectively stratify patients based on the major variables of interest (procedures, tests, comorbidities, etc.), or alternatively, multiple trials should each focus on a specific aspect of the research question. In particular, since it is likely that the effect of preoperative testing will vary substantially based on the specific surgery (as suggested by the different effects found between cataract trials and general surgery studies), trials should either focus on a single type of surgery or, at a minimum, stratify their results by surgery or surgery risk class. Furthermore, studies should stratify their results based on patient risk category, such as ASA category and comorbidities. Studies should capture the full range of perioperative outcomes, including patient quality of life/satisfaction and resource utilization. Studies should be sufficiently powered to evaluate, at a minimum, total major perioperative complications. Preferably they should be sufficiently powered to cover specific major complications, such as death. Also, preferably they should be sufficiently powered to allow for a priori subgroup analyses and analyses specific to at least some individual procedures and tests.

Observational studies can provide a lesser level of evidence to provide information on the comparative effectiveness of alternative preoperative testing strategies. However, the intrinsic heterogeneity and risk of confounding require that great care and attention be given to how the data are analyzed (e.g., with a priori subgroup analyses) and whether it is possible to adequately adjust for fundamental differences between nonrandomized cohorts of patients having or not having testing done. At a minimum, observational studies need to be adjusted for differences in patient and surgical characteristics and to control for cluster effects for individual surgeons or based on surgical experience. To be of use, observational studies should include concurrent patients who do or do not receive testing and who are as similar as possible. Even then, it will be important to use strong statistical methods to adjust analyses for differences in the cohorts unrelated to testing and confounders (e.g., propensity score or instrumental variable methods). All the suggestions made for RCTs regarding focusing or stratifying analyses based on surgical, patient, and other study characteristics also apply to observational studies.

In the face of a paucity of reliable evidence regarding the benefits, harms, and resources used with routine or per-protocol preoperative testing, decision analyses may be of value to delineate plausible estimates of the range of how beneficial or harmful and resource intensive preoperative testing could be. Such analyses could be useful to rank tests and procedures by likely benefit and thus help to prioritize research for specific tests and procedures. Such models will require direct evidence of the comparative effect of testing, as reviewed here, along with other indirect evidence, including the likelihood of specific perioperative complications for specific procedures, the likelihood that specific tests would diagnose conditions that would impact the rate of complications, the effects of correcting or ameliorating any such conditions, whether a test result could be acted on to impact the rate of complications, the likelihood of true- and false-positive test results, and the effects of delaying or canceling the procedures.

Regardless of the design of future studies, to allow answers about the value of routine or per-protocol preoperative testing, it is important that a large number of studies be conducted covering a wide range of scenarios, but that they be specific enough to allow applicability to decisionmaking for particular patients undergoing particular procedures in a given setting. Alternative prioritization approaches may be reasonable. Initially focusing on people who are most likely to have life-threatening perioperative complications, including older patients, those in higher ASA categories, those with important comorbidities, and those undergoing higher risk surgeries, would allow for relatively small, low-resource studies that would be adequately powered. In these cases, complications would be more common and test abnormalities may also be more common. Not only would studies of these groups have the greatest potential to affect patients most likely to have complications, but the studies would also be better powered due to the higher complication rates than in lower risk populations. Further studies of patients at high risk of surgical bleeding (for example, children undergoing tonsillectomy and/or adenoidectomy) are also warranted. Alternatively, one could argue that future research should focus on lower risk populations and surgeries. While these studies would need to be relatively large due to low complication rates, the findings of these studies may have the greatest impact since they would address more common surgeries and more typical patients. Furthermore, hospitals, clinicians, and patients may be more willing to forgo preoperative testing in low- rather than high-risk settings. We believe it is likely that higher risk patients undergoing higher risk procedures would continue to have preoperative testing done regardless of evidence showing the testing to be ineffective. Given the different arguments that could be made about who to include in future studies and limited resources to conduct such research, this topic may be worthy of undergoing a formal value-of-information analysis.[10]

Conclusions

With the exception of cataract surgery, there is a paucity of reliable evidence regarding the benefits, harms, and resource utilization associated with routine or per-protocol preoperative testing for all tests used for all procedures. There is a high strength of evidence, which is broadly applicable, that ECG, basic metabolic panel (biochemistry), and CBC have no effect on important clinical outcomes in patients scheduled for cataract surgery, including total perioperative complications and procedure cancellations. But despite several nonrandomized studies, there is insufficient evidence regarding the value of routine or per-protocol preoperative testing for other procedures and populations. Based on studies with a high risk of bias, there is a possibility that complications and deaths occurred more commonly among patients undergoing ad hoc as opposed to routine or per-protocol testing. This raises a caution against extrapolating the cataract findings to other surgeries and populations who may be at higher risk of complications due to the nature of the procedures or underlying illnesses and comorbidities. The evidence is insufficient to clarify specifically which routinely conducted or per-protocol tests may be of benefit or no benefit for which patients undergoing which procedures. There is no evidence regarding quality of life or satisfaction, resource utilization, or harms of testing. There is also no evidence regarding how the value of testing may differ based on the risks of a specific surgical procedure; the type of anesthesia planned; the indication for surgery; comorbidities or other patient characteristics; the structure of testing (e.g., routine for everyone vs. per protocol, whether testing is conducted in a specialized preoperative clinic); who orders the tests (e.g., surgeon vs. anesthesiologist vs. primary care physician); or the length of time prior to the procedure that the tests are conducted. Given the large number of patients undergoing elective surgery, there is a clear need to develop better evidence for when routine or per-protocol testing improves patient outcomes and what the harms may be.

References

1. Apfelbaum JL, Connis RT, Nickinovich DG, et al. Practice advisory for preanesthesia evaluation: an updated report by the American Society of Anesthesiologists Task Force on Preanesthesia Evaluation. Anesthesiology. 2012 Mar;116(3):522-38. PMID: 22273990.

2. Kumar A, Srivastava U. Role of routine laboratory investigations in preoperative evaluation. J Anaesthesiol Clin Pharmacol. 2011 Apr;27(2):174-9. PMID: 21772675.

3. Bryson GL. Has preoperative testing become a habit? Can J Anaesth. 2005 Jun;52(6):557-61. PMID: 15983138.

4. Kaplan EB, Sheiner LB, Boeckmann AJ, et al. The usefulness of preoperative laboratory screening. JAMA. 1985 Jun 28;253(24):3576-81. PMID: 3999339.

5. Johnson RK, Mortimer AJ. Routine pre-operative blood testing: is it necessary? Anaesthesia. 2002 Sep;57(9):914-7. PMID: 12190758.

6. Pasternak LR. Preoperative testing: moving from individual testing to risk management. Anesth Analg. 2009 Feb;108(2):393-4. PMID: 19151262.

7. MacPherson RD, Reeve SA, Stewart TV, et al. Effective strategy to guide pathology test ordering in surgical patients. ANZ J Surg. 2005 Mar;75(3):138-43. PMID: 15777393.

8. Klein AA, Arrowsmith JE. Should routine pre-operative testing be abandoned? Anaesthesia. 2010 Oct;65(10):974-6. PMID: 21198466.

9. Methods Guide for Effectiveness and Comparative Effectiveness Reviews. AHRQ Publication No. 10(11)-EHC063-EF. Rockville, MD: Agency for Healthcare Research and Quality; March 2011. Chapters available at www.effectivehealthcare.ahrq.gov.

10. Myers E, Sanders GD, Ravi D, et al. Evaluating the Potential Use of Modeling and Value-of-Information Analysis for Future Research Prioritization Within the Evidence-based Practice Center Program. (Prepared by the Duke Evidence-based Practice Center under Contract No. 290-2007-10066-I.) AHRQ Publication No. 11-EHC030-EF. Rockville, MD: Agency for Healthcare Research and Quality. June 2011. www.effectivehealthcare.ahrq.gov/reports/final.cfm.

Introduction

Traditionally, preoperative testing has been part of the preoperative care process to inform patient selection by determining fitness for anesthesia and identifying patients at high risk for perioperative complications. Routine preoperative tests are defined by the American Society of Anesthesiologists (ASA) as those done in the absence of any specific clinical indication or purpose and typically include a panel of blood tests, urine tests, chest radiography, and electrocardiogram (ECG).[1,2] These tests are performed to find latent abnormalities, such as anemia or silent heart disease, that could impact how, when, or whether the planned surgical procedure and concomitant anesthesia are performed. Tests performed either to assess the condition for which the procedure is being performed (e.g., visual acuity testing prior to cataract surgery) or to plan the surgery (e.g., imaging tests prior to cancer excision) are not considered routine preoperative testing.

Many hospitals have instituted protocols to perform a series of laboratory tests prior to any operative procedure under the assumption that this information will enhance safety for surgical patients and reduce liability for adverse events.[2] During the past three decades routine preoperative testing has been challenged by several academic publications with concerns about the sizable cost of testing, overtesting and the consequences of false positive tests (leading to unnecessary workups and treatments), and the unknown benefit to patients.[3-8] Preoperative testing is estimated to cost the U.S. $18 billion annually.[2] In addition to increasing the cost of surgical care,[2] nonselective preoperative testing may result in false positive or borderline results (in the absence of clinical indication), which require further investigation. Additional investigation may cause unnecessary psychological and economic burdens, postponement of surgery, and even morbidity and mortality (e.g., complications due to unnecessary biopsies performed to follow up false positive laboratory tests).[2] As all routine testing does, preoperative testing will find some abnormal test results that will lead to new diagnoses (such as previously undetected lung cancer), but it is unclear whether the benefits of identifying and treating unsuspected abnormalities outweigh the harms of false positive preoperative tests and, if there is a net benefit, how this benefit compares to the resource utilization required for testing.

Three professional medical associations nominated this topic for systematic review, citing the wide variation in clinical practice, the need for a guideline for routine preoperative testing, and the likelihood that a comparative effectiveness review on this subject would have broad clinical impact—particularly if such a review included the most commonly ordered tests in healthy patients, as well as those with comorbidities, undergoing a wide variety of high- and low-risk surgeries.

Since the UK's National Institute for Health and Clinical Excellence (NICE) published an evidence-based review and guideline titled "The Use of Routine Preoperative Tests for Elective Surgery" in 2003,[9] there have been no other systematic reviews, including AHRQ reports, comprehensively covering this topic. A subsequent Health Technology Assessment conducted a limited systematic review in 2008 (published in 2012) of blood and pulmonary function tests in low- or medium-risk patients,[10] but they included no studies comparing testing versus no testing. A recent Cochrane review focused on randomized controlled trials (RCTs) of routine preoperative testing for cataract surgery. It concluded that there is no increase in safety of cataract surgery with routine preoperative testing.[11] The American College of Cardiology and the American Heart Association (ACC/AHA) published a guideline on perioperative cardiovascular evaluation in 2007,[12] which in part covered routine preoperative tests prior to cardiovascular surgery and routine preoperative cardiovascular tests (e.g., transesophageal echocardiography) for noncardiovascular surgery, but their review was considerably narrower in scope than this review.

The ACC/AHA guidelines help ascertain cardiac risk in patients undergoing noncardiac surgery. A consistent theme is that routine cardiac testing is rarely indicated and that intervention rarely lowers the risk of a procedure unless the intervention was indicated irrespective of the patient's upcoming surgery. For example, the ACC/AHA guidelines state that ECG is not indicated for asymptomatic patients undergoing low risk surgery. The American College of Radiology published Appropriateness Criteria (last reviewed in 2011) for chest radiography, which, similar to the ACC/AHA guidelines, state that routine chest radiography in asymptomatic patients is usually not appropriate and exposes patient to unnecessary radiation.[13] The ASA likewise published a practice advisory in 2012, which stated that preoperative testing should not be ordered routinely, but acknowledged insufficient evidence to identify explicit rules for ordering preoperative tests based on specific clinical characteristics.[1]

Considerations for the Evaluation of Preoperative Testing

Alternative Testing Strategies

There is no common terminology among anesthesiologists and surgeons regarding the alternative preoperative testing strategies. For this review, we use the terms routine, per protocol, and or ad hoc as defined here:

1. Routine preoperative testing, where the tests of interest are conducted in all patients undergoing a given procedure, regardless of medical history or other patient features. Common examples of this approach are coagulation studies for all patients undergoing tonsillectomy or routine hematocrit levels for all patients undergoing surgeries with any expected blood loss.
2. Per protocol preoperative testing, where the tests of interest are conducted in a predefined subset of patients undergoing a given procedure. Implicitly or explicitly, the patients chosen for testing are those who, as a group, are considered to be at above-average risk for procedure-related complications. Common criteria used are age, medical history, and anesthesia or surgical risk category. Specific examples include obtaining electrocardiograms (ECGs) in all patients 50 years or older or kidney function tests in patients who have diabetes or are taking certain medications.
3. Ad hoc (or elective) testing, where preoperative testing is done at the discretion of the clinician doing a preoperative evaluation, based on patient history and physical examination (H&P) findings. No tests are done routinely or based on any protocol. The reasons for obtaining (or foregoing) a test will vary widely across patients and across ordering clinicians.

A fourth alternative, not explicitly considered here, would be a policy proscribing any testing prior to surgery. While this approach may theoretically be an option, it is not a real-world alternative in high-income countries.

In practice (and in research studies) there may also be overlap or combinations of these alternatives. A protocol may require that some tests be performed in all patients (e.g., complete blood counts [CBC]) but other tests be performed per protocol. Of course, in almost all settings, clinicians will have the option to add ad hoc tests to a list of routine or per protocol tests.

Preoperative Tests

There are many preoperative tests that can be ordered for a patient and will help determine fitness for surgery and anesthesia. Routine tests are those that may be of value to reduce the risk of procedural complications but are not directly related to the planned procedure. The specific tests under review here are listed in the Methods section and include hematologic, metabolic, and organ function blood tests, hemostasis tests, urinalysis, chest radiography (and related tests), ECG (and related tests), and pregnancy tests. These tests may be done alone (e.g., only a pregnancy test) or as a panel of tests. Since different tests evaluate different conditions with different levels of accuracy, they can be expected to predict different complications and to be of varying value for different patients undergoing different procedures.

Patient and Procedure Heterogeneity

Patients undergoing surgery show considerable variation in demographic characteristics, underlying health and comorbidities, indications for surgery, specific surgery planned, type of anesthesia planned (e.g., general versus spinal anesthesia), and other factors. Differences among these factors may result in differences in the benefits of finding abnormalities (e.g., anemia) and in the potential harms of testing (e.g., delayed surgery or unnecessary colonoscopy). Therefore, it is important to look not only at the benefits and harms of preoperative testing in general, but also at specific patient and intervention (surgery-related) factors that might change the balance between the benefits and harms; namely the risk of the surgical procedure, type of anesthesia planned, indication for surgery, comorbidities, and other patient characteristics.

Surgical Procedures

The risk of procedural complications varies widely based on the type of surgery. It thus follows that the potential benefit of preoperative testing will vary based on the risk of complications related to the planned surgery. While there is not a widely used methodology for determining overall surgical risk, we provide an example of a simple categorization, used effectively by the 2003 NICE guideline,[9] which grades surgeries by the complexity and likelihood of blood loss and complications (Table 1). Other surgical risk categorizations have been developed, but are generally less generalizable. For example, the American College of Cardiology/American Heart Association Task Force on Practice Guidelines ranked procedures as high, medium, and low based on cardiac risk.[12] Although it has yet to be demonstrated, one could expect that some preoperative tests may be of greater value in reducing complications in higher- rather than lower risk surgeries.

Table 1. Surgical severity grades, from 2003 NICE guideline[9]

Grade	Procedure Examples
Grade 1 (minor)	Cataract excision Skin lesion excision Breast abscess drainage
Grade 2 (intermediate)	Inguinal hernia primary repair Varicose vein excision Tonsillectomy/adenoidectomy Knee arthroscopy
Grade 3 (major)	Total abdominal hysterectomy Lumbar discectomy
Grade 4 (major+)	Total joint replacement Lung surgery Colonic resection Radical neck dissection Neurosurgery Cardiac surgery

Patient Health Status

Similarly, one could expect that the risk of complications, and thus the potential value of preoperative testing, may be greater for patients with worse overall health status. The American Society of Anesthesiologists (ASA) physical status classification system was created to assess a patient's fitness for surgery. The six categories are listed in Table 2. ASA class is commonly assessed and reported, and it may be an important factor in determining which patients would most benefit from preoperative testing (i.e., which patients should be included in a testing protocol). However, it should be noted that there is no explicit definition for each of the status classes; thus the categorization of individual patients into different classes may vary widely from hospital to hospital and anesthesiologist to anesthesiologist.

Table 2. American Society of Anesthesiologists (ASA) physical status classification system[14]

Class	Definition
ASA Physical Status 1	A normal healthy patient
ASA Physical Status 2	A patient with mild systemic disease
ASA Physical Status 3	A patient with severe systemic disease
ASA Physical Status 4	A patient with severe systemic disease that is a constant threat to life
ASA Physical Status 5	A moribund patient who is not expected to survive without the operation
ASA Physical Status 6	A declared brain-dead patient whose organs are being removed for donor purposes

Patient Clinical Characteristics

Beyond ASA class, patients undergoing surgery have considerable variation in clinical characteristics. This variation may lead to substantial differences in how abnormal preoperative testing findings are handled, as well as their potential effect on surgery. For example, an abnormal ECG performed as part of a protocol in a patient with history of coronary artery disease may result in a different preoperative intervention or a different threshold for canceling surgery than in a patient with no cardiac history, risk factors, or symptoms.

Anesthesia Type

In general, preoperative testing is considered primarily for procedures that require a member of an anesthetic team (anesthesiologist, certified registered nurse anesthetist, or equivalent). The type of anesthesia used is determined by the complexity and invasiveness of the planned surgery, the patient's medical condition and history, and his or her preferences. Types of anesthesia include general anesthesia, monitored anesthesia care (MAC, also known as sedation anesthesia or local anesthesia with sedation), neuraxial anesthesia (spinal or epidural), or regional anesthesia, including peripheral nerve block (such as femoral or brachial plexus blocks) or intravenous regional anesthesia (Bier block). Preprocedure testing is generally of limited utility for procedures requiring only local anesthesia or only sedation (without anesthesia). Different anesthetic techniques carry different risks and rates of complications; thus, preoperative testing may be of different value for patients undergoing different types of anesthesia. However, as noted, the type of anesthesia will be confounded with the type of surgery and the patient's medical condition.

Clinician- and Setting-Based Differences

Inefficiencies in the preoperative testing processes or failures in the handoff of test results between primary care physicians, surgeons, and anesthesiologists ultimately affect the clinical utility of preoperative testing. Different hospitals, surgeons, and anesthesiologists have different protocols for preoperative testing, including, but not limited to, ad hoc testing by the surgeon or anesthesiologist, referral to the patient's primary care physician for testing at his or her discretion, and dedicated clinics with standardized protocols based on a patient's health status and planned surgery. Further, the comparator intervention, ad hoc testing, is by definition variable, depending on the clinician ordering the test, to what degree testing is based on any H&P he or she performs, and each clinician's likelihood of ordering few or many tests, which in part will be based on the local culture. Subsequent to testing, there is an implementation issue, in that any changes to patient outcomes due to testing must be mediated through clinical decisions about how to act on abnormal tests. Again, individual clinicians, different specialties, and different surgical settings are likely to have different thresholds for when and how to respond to abnormal tests. Examples include decisions about whether to delay or cancel surgery or whether to administer blood components preoperatively. This variability in care practices raises questions about whether ad hoc testing results in under- and/or over-utilization of tests (balancing benefits and harms) compared with per protocol testing, as well as whether testing ordered and followed up by different disciplines or types of clinicians have equivalent clinical utility. Examples of potentially ineffective testing due to process failures include tests performed by primary care physicians that are not transmitted to or followed up by surgeons and tests done by anesthesiologists that are not transmitted to or followed up by primary care physicians. There remains a lack of knowledge as to whether patient outcomes differ based on differences in testing protocols.

Timing of Testing

A final factor that needs to be considered is the timing of the tests. Hospitals or surgical centers may dictate that preoperative testing must be done within a limited period of time before surgery, such as 30 days or 6 months. Anecdotally, this results in changes in surgical practice, such as performing the second eye cataract surgery earlier than would otherwise be indicated so that preoperative testing does not have to be repeated. However, it is unknown whether there is adequate evidence to support any particular time threshold for preoperative tests.

Assessing the Clinical Utility of Preoperative Testing

Preoperative testing can have a direct impact only on certain outcomes of interest, including emotional and cognitive changes in the patient conferred by testing and its results, any harms associated with the testing procedure (e.g., pain, hemorrhage, or bruising from a blood draw, exposure to ionizing radiation from imaging tests), and costs to the patient (in the form of time spent or copayments) or other types of resource utilization. For the most part, however, testing has indirect effects:

- Test results can influence treatment choices, such as managing the abnormal test result (e.g., by blood transfusion) or changing the surgical or anesthetic technique (e.g., changing from general to regional anesthesia), and through them, patient outcomes (e.g., a previously unknown test abnormality may confer an increased risk of surgical mortality; the surgery thus may be appropriately delayed or canceled)
- Testing can prolong time to the procedure for logistical reasons (either appropriately to allow correction of or further treatment due to the abnormal test result or unnecessarily if no further treatment or evaluation was truly needed)
- Abnormal test results may lead to cascade testing (either appropriately if the test result signals a real abnormality or unnecessarily if the test result was spurious or was not due to a clinically important abnormality)

Therefore, when assessing the clinical effects of testing, we need to assess the clinical utility of patient-management strategies that include the testing and its downstream indirect effects. At the systems level, the volume of testing has a direct impact on resource utilization and costs borne by patients and payers. Further, unnecessary testing can overload resources with limited bandwidth (e.g., imaging), representing at a minimum an increase in managing and scheduling overhead.

Comparative studies (comparing different preoperative testing strategies) can effectively analyze all outcomes of interest. The range of outcomes that can be meaningfully assessed by noncomparative (cohort) studies, though, is more limited. Complication rates, the most important patient-centered outcomes, can only be adequately assessed by comparative studies, since the underlying risk of complications will vary across cohorts of patients and types of surgery. The complication rate in a cohort study of routine testing is difficult to interpret without an estimate of the expected complication rate without routine testing. The only outcomes from cohort studies that can provide some information to address the Key Questions are those directly related to the testing, such as surgery cancelation or delay due to an abnormal test. However, this outcome is of somewhat limited value since it does not address whether the patient was benefited or harmed by the surgical cancelation or delay.

Statement of Work

In 2011, nominators proposed questions related to routine preoperative testing to AHRQ to form the basis of a comparative effectiveness review. The topic went through a process of topic refinement with a panel of Key Informants (including domain experts in anesthesia, general and breast surgery, and cardiology; health care payers with an interest in preoperative testing; a patient advocate; and representatives from the three nominators) and local domain experts (including an epidemiologist, internist, anesthesiologist, ophthalmologist, radiologist, and a thoracic and general surgeon). As described further in the Methods section, we also convened a Technical Expert Panel (TEP) to finalize the protocol. These panels generally agreed that the primary questions of interest related to the effectiveness of performing routine preoperative testing on a broad range of patients scheduled for a broad range of procedures requiring anesthesia with a variety of tests. The target audience for this review includes surgeons, anesthesiologists, and other clinicians involved in perioperative care of surgical patients; policymakers, including clinical practice guideline developers and surgical clinic administrators involved in determining preoperative testing policies and protocols; healthcare payers; researchers with an interest in perioperative care; and, ultimately, patients undergoing surgical procedures. While there was some discussion of limiting the range of procedures to either exclude "high risk" elective surgeries (given the existence of guidance for these surgeries related to cardiac risk from the ACC/AHA [12]) or to the most common surgeries in the U.S., it was ultimately agreed to keep a broad purview. Furthermore, since anesthesia is commonly used for some nonsurgical procedures (such as electroconvulsive therapy) and thus preoperative testing may be considered, it was agreed to include both surgical and nonsurgical procedures that require the presence of an anesthetist (i.e., excluding sedation alone). The stakeholder panels also reviewed various lists of potential tests to be considered. The most complete list considered was from the NICE evidence-based review and guideline.[9] While some tests were considered for exclusion, ultimately it was agreed to include a broad range of tests, based primarily on the tests that have been examined in studies. The final list of included tests is in the Methods section. After a series of discussions about what research questions would provide solid evidence about the actual value of routine (or per protocol) preoperative testing to reduce perioperative complications, as opposed to evidence that would support the contention that testing could theoretically reduce these complications, it was agreed to limit the scope of the key questions. The decision to focus this review on direct evidence (evidence regarding actual changes in patient outcomes and management) was made in part due to time and resource constraints. The restrictions to the scope of the Key Questions are described further in the following section.

This Comparative Effectiveness Review analyzes the value of routine and per protocol preoperative testing in patients undergoing procedures requiring anesthesia or sedation. The review focuses on the direct evidence of the comparative value of routine preoperative testing versus not testing (or other protocols for testing). This evidence is derived primarily from studies that directly compare testing protocols. These are the only studies that can demonstrate whether uniformly testing an unselected population prior to surgery leads to better outcomes for those patients. We also include cohort studies that report rates of "process outcomes" (rates of surgery cancellation, changes to planned surgery or anesthesia, etc.) only for patients being tested since the rate of procedure delay and cancellation, etc., due to testing is, by definition, zero in patients who do not undergo testing. However, no implicit comparison can be made with patients who undergo ad hoc testing based on their H&P.

The review does not evaluate questions that, while important and related to the topic at hand, do not provide direct evidence of the comparative value of testing versus not testing. The review does not evaluate analyses that would require assumptions about what might have occurred without testing (e.g., studies that reported complications only in patients who underwent testing) or assumptions about how testing might improve outcomes based on different rates of complications among patients with abnormal and normal preoperative tests. Specifically,

1. We do not assess the benefits and harms of preoperative testing based on the incidence of: perioperative complications (such as major bleeding) in studies that report only on patients who underwent testing (i.e., noncomparative studies). Two examples of such an analysis would be 1) a study that found no perioperative cardiac events and thus concluded that a preoperative electrocardiogram (ECG) would not have been of value; and 2) a study that found potentially preventable episodes of clinically significant postoperative bleeding and thus concluded that a preoperative bleeding time test would

have been of value. While these studies make conclusions regarding the possible value of testing, they do not provide evidence regarding the actual effect of routine preoperative tests since the complication rates absent routine testing is unknown.

2. We do not systematically review the prevalence rates of abnormal test results for different populations of patients undergoing surgery. Some studies have reported that, because a given percentage of patients have an abnormal preoperative test (such as a chest radiograph) and the surgical and anesthesia teams could alter their care based on these abnormalities, patients could benefit from the test. However, such studies again do not provide evidence that actually ordering the test would alter perioperative outcomes since the effect of acting on the abnormal test result on perioperative outcomes is unknown.

3. We do not systematically review the test performance (e.g., sensitivity and specificity) of any of the tests. To systematically review test performance would require a broader review of each test, beyond its use in routine preoperative testing, than would be required to answer the given key questions. Further, test performance without patient outcomes does not directly address the value of routine preoperative testing; the effect of acting on the (true or false) abnormal test result on perioperative outcomes is unknown.

4. We do not assesses test results (i.e., abnormal vs. normal test results) as predictors of outcomes. The goal of this review is to assess whether actually ordering routine preoperative tests alters care and patient outcomes. We are not evaluating the predictors of clinical outcomes, including abnormal test results; association studies do not provide data on how the test performs in different populations or the balance of benefits and harms. For example, we do not evaluate whether patients with abnormal ECGs are at higher risk of perioperative complications than patients with normal ECGs. Instead, we evaluate whether patients who had ECGs performed routinely had different outcomes than patients who did not.

These types of analyses are too indirect to the questions at hand and would not provide convincing evidence regarding the comparative effectiveness of routine or per protocol testing versus ad hoc or no testing. Also, since the impact of testing is mediated by management change, abnormal test results that are not or cannot be acted on will not prevent perioperative complications. This review is focused on addressing, as best possible, the direct, comparative evidence. However, in the Future Research section of the Discussion, we discuss how indirect evidence could be incorporated in decision modeling.

Analytic Framework

To guide the development of the Key Questions for the evaluation of preoperative testing, we developed an analytic framework (Figure 1) that maps the specific linkages associating the populations of interest, the interventions, the outcomes of interest (including harms), and the potential modifying factors. Specifically, this analytic framework depicts the chain of logic that the evidence must support to link the interventions to improved health outcomes.

Figure 1. Analytic framework for routine preoperative testing

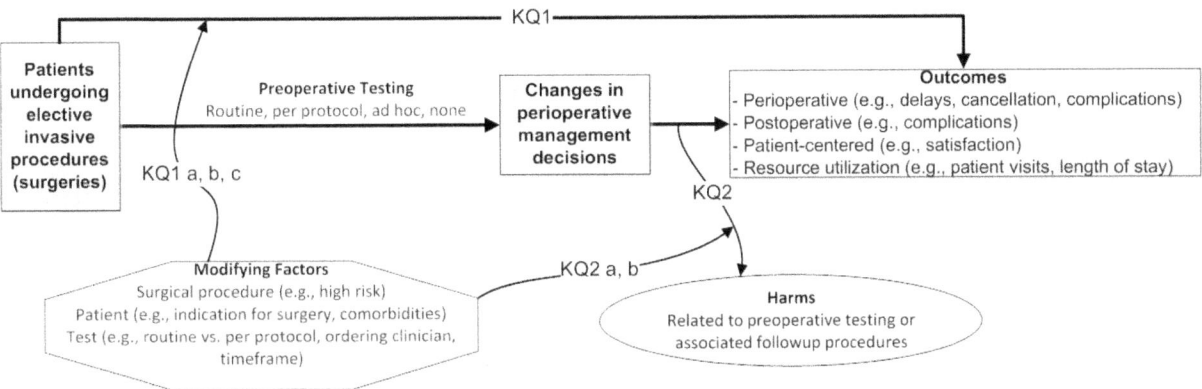

KQ = Key Question.

Key Questions

Key Question 1: How do routine or per protocol preoperative testing strategies compare to no testing or alternative testing strategies with respect to outcomes—including perioperative clinical outcomes, quality of life or satisfaction, periprocedural patient management decisions, and resource utilization—among patients undergoing elective surgical procedures? How do outcomes vary by:

    a. the risk of the surgical procedure, the type of anesthesia planned, the indication for surgery, comorbidities, or other patient characteristics

    b. the structure of testing (e.g., routine for everyone vs. per protocol, whether testing is conducted in a specialized preoperative clinic) or by who orders the tests (e.g., surgeon vs. anesthesiologist vs. primary care physician)

    c. the length of time prior to the procedure that the tests are conducted

Key Question 2: What are the harms of routine or per protocol preoperative testing strategies compared to no testing or to an alternative testing strategies? How do outcomes vary by:

    a. the risk of the surgical procedure, the type of anesthesia planned, the indication for surgery, comorbidities, or other patient characteristics

    b. the structure of testing (e.g., routine for everyone vs. per protocol, whether testing is conducted in a specialized preoperative clinic) or by who orders the tests (e.g., surgeon vs. anesthesiologist vs. primary care physician)

Methods

The present Comparative Effectiveness Review (CER) follows the methodology outlined in the Agency for Healthcare Research and Quality's (AHRQ) 2012 "Methods Guide for Effectiveness and Comparative Effectiveness Reviews," available at http://effectivehealthcare.ahrq.gov/ehc/products/60/318/MethodsGuide_Prepublication-Draft_20120523.pdf.

AHRQ Task Order Officer

The AHRQ Task Order Officer (TOO) was responsible for overseeing all aspects of this project. The TOO facilitated a common understanding among all parties involved in the project, resolved ambiguities, and fielded all Evidence-based Practice Center (EPC) queries regarding the scope and processes of the project. The TOO and other staff at AHRQ helped to establish the Key Questions and protocol and reviewed the report for consistency, clarity, and to ensure that it conforms to AHRQ standards.

External Expert Input

During a topic refinement phase, the questions that had initially been nominated for this report were refined with input from a panel of Key Informants. The Key Informants included experts in anesthesia, general surgery, thoracic surgery, ophthalmology, radiology, internal medicine, and epidemiology. After a public review of the proposed Key Questions, a new panel of experts was convened to form the TEP. The TEP included experts in anesthesia, general surgery, urology, cardiology, internal medicine, and family medicine. The TEP provided input to help refine the protocol, identify important issues, and define the parameters for the review of evidence. The TEP was also asked to suggest additional studies.

Literature Search

We conducted literature searches of studies in MEDLINE® and Ovid Healthstar® (inception – 22 July 2013), as well as the Cochrane Central Trials Registry® and Cochrane Database of Systematic Reviews® (through 2nd Quarter, 2013). The reference lists of prior systematic reviews and relevant guidelines were hand-searched. All citations were screened to identify articles relevant to each Key Question. The search included terms for surgical procedures, preoperative care, diagnostic tests, including the specific tests ECG, chest radiography, blood counts, coagulation tests, biochemistry, glucose, urinalysis, kidney function tests, liver function tests, pregnancy tests, hemoglobinopathies, and pulmonary function tests (see Appendix A for complete search strings).

Scientific Information Packets were not solicited from industry, professional societies, or other interested researchers because all the tests have been in use for a long time and additional proprietary information is unlikely.

Study Selection and Eligibility Criteria

The EPC has developed a computerized screening program, *Abstrackr*, to automate the screening of abstracts for eligible articles for full-text screening (http://sunfire34.eecs.tufts.edu).[15] Three team members double-screened all abstracts after an iterative training period to ensure that all screeners agreed upon the eligibility criteria. *Abstrackr* allowed us to label each citation as "accept," "reject," or "maybe." All abstracts with disagreements between readers or labeled as "maybe" were reconciled by the whole team in conference.

Full-text articles were retrieved for all potentially relevant articles. These were rescreened for eligibility. All rejected articles were confirmed by the team leader. The reasons for excluding these articles are tabulated in Appendix B.

Study eligibility was based on the following selection criteria: population and surgical procedure of interest, interventions (i.e., tests) and comparators of interest, outcomes of interest, and study designs. We did not consider outcomes when conducting abstract screening.

Population and Condition of Interest

We included studies conducted in both adults (≥18 years) and children undergoing surgical procedures requiring either anesthesia or sedation. This included
- Patients undergoing any elective or ambulatory surgical or other invasive procedure that commonly requires anesthesia or sedation of any type or approach that is administered by an anesthesia team member. Cataract surgery was included regardless of local practice regarding anesthesia or sedation.
- Procedures in any setting, including inpatient, outpatient, and office-based.
- Any category of risk for surgical or anesthetic complications.
- Surgical procedures in any risk category, ranging from minor and minimally invasive through high risk, maximally invasive surgeries (e.g., vascular, neurologic, thoracic, abdominal, and pelvic surgeries).
- Patients undergoing nonsurgical diagnostic procedures that may require anesthesia or sedation (e.g., biopsy, colonoscopy) were excluded.

Interventions of Interest

We included all preoperative tests likely to be conducted routinely (or on a per protocol basis). These included basic laboratory tests, simple radiography, and selective other relatively simple diagnostic tests.

We included:
- Electrolytes (e.g., sodium, potassium, bicarbonate, chloride)
- Kidney function tests (e.g., blood urea nitrogen, creatinine, glomerular filtration rate)
- Liver function tests (or other components of a "complete metabolic panel")
- Glycemia measures (e.g., glucose, hemoglobin A1c)
- Blood counts (e.g., hemoglobin, hematocrit, white blood cells, platelets)
- Bleeding and coagulation tests (e.g., prothrombin time, bleeding test)
- Hemoglobinopathy tests (e.g., sickle cell)
- Urinalysis
- Pregnancy tests

- Chest radiography
- Electrocardiograms (ECG), 12 lead
- Cardiac stress tests
- Basic echocardiogram
- Pulmonary function tests

Other tests of potential interest were considered on a case-by-case basis and discussed with the TEP prior to inclusion. We excluded costly and invasive testing since these are not routinely performed in all patients or in a large group of patients per protocol or are used only in highly selective patients. Examples of excluded tests were computed tomography and magnetic resonance imaging tests, tests requiring markers or dyes (e.g., thallium stress testing), and invasive tests (e.g., angiography).

The tests had to have been conducted in the preoperative period (although we did not apply a maximum duration of time prior to the surgical procedure). At least implicitly, the tests had to have been performed for the purpose of assessing the patient's risk and status prior to the planned procedure. We excluded tests performed for the purpose of diagnosis or staging the disease for which the surgery was being performed or for specific surgical planning (e.g., imaging tests to determine the extent of cancer or echocardiography to evaluate valvular dysfunction prior to cardiac surgery). We also excluded patient factors other than tests, including patient history, symptoms, physical examination signs or findings, and demographic features, or panels of "tests" that included any of these factors. While patient symptoms, such as decompensated congestive heart failure, may be important reasons for altering, delaying, or canceling surgery, these should be routinely assessed as part of an appropriate standard of care.

In addition, for a given surgical procedure (or set of procedures), the tests had to have been conducted either routinely (i.e., in all patients undergoing the procedure, regardless of age, sex, or medical condition) or based on a standard protocol (i.e., in all patients who met certain predetermined criteria based on age, sex, medical condition, or other factors).

Intervention and comparator arms were sorted into four categories: routine (everyone was scheduled to have all tests), per protocol (a protocol was used to determine who had which tests), ad hoc (testing was done at a clinician's discretion), or no testing. The distinction between routine and per protocol testing was not always clear. If a study did not report sufficient information to distinguish the two, we assumed that routine testing was conducted. In a few instances, when a large number of tests were done routinely and a single test (e.g., ECG) was done per protocol, we also categorized this as routine testing.

Comparators of Interest

Comparators of interest included no preoperative testing (of a panel of tests or by individual test), "ad hoc" testing (i.e., the tests were conducted at the discretion of the ordering clinician, regardless of the reason), per protocol testing (as a comparator to routine testing), a different panel of routine tests, testing conducted in a different setting or by a different type of clinician (e.g., in a specialized preoperative testing clinic versus by the patient's primary care physician), and testing done at different presurgery time points (e.g., within 30 days vs. within 6 months).

Outcomes of Interest

For Key Question 1, outcomes of interest included clinical, other patient-centered, and intermediate outcomes. The outcomes were confined to those related to the conduct of the surgical procedures and anesthesia, perioperative events, patient satisfaction, and resource utilization. Specifically, these included:

- Clinical and other patient-centered outcomes
  - Procedure or anesthesia delay
  - Procedure cancellation
  - Perioperative clinical outcomes
    - Mortality
    - Surgical complications
  - Patient quality of life
  - Patient satisfaction
  - Patient resources, including time and lost work
  - Unplanned hospital admission or readmission within 30 days
  - Change in disposition of care (e.g., unplanned intensive care unit admission)
  - Length of hospital stay
  - Other resource utilization, including unplanned followup tests or procedures
- Intermediate outcome
  - Changes to perioperative patient management (other than procedure delay or cancellation)

For Key Question 2, outcomes of interest included adverse events or harms related to testing. Specifically, these included:

- Unnecessary or inappropriate procedure or anesthesia delays (based on an adjudication decision regarding appropriateness)
- Unnecessary or inappropriate procedure cancellation (based on an adjudication decision regarding appropriateness)
- Harms from testing or from interventions that resulted from test results
- "Unnecessary" followup tests or procedures (i.e., negative followup tests suggesting the preoperative test was false positive; e.g., a normal chest CT performed as followup to an abnormal routine preoperative chest radiography)

Eligible Study Designs

We included published, peer-reviewed articles. We included studies in any patient setting where testing or surgical procedures may be conducted, including hospitals, inpatient and outpatient clinics, and clinicians' offices. We included studies that covered any timeframe, although they had to be longitudinal in design to the extent that testing was done prior to the planned procedure and followup occurred at least to the time of the procedure.

We included comparative studies (in which one or more protocols for testing was compared with other protocols for testing, including protocols for no testing), whether randomized or not. We included both prospective and retrospective studies. Eligible retrospective studies must have clearly included a sample of patients who received routine preoperative testing, not just patients who had preoperative testing done on an ad hoc basis. These could have included pre-post studies (e.g., before or after a testing policy was implemented) or studies with historical controls (where current practice is compared with a prior period at the same or a different institution).

Because we expected the comparative studies to be limited in quantity and quality, we also evaluated cohort (noncomparative, single group studies in which all study participants had the same testing battery or protocol). However, we limited these studies to those that reported "process" outcomes where the process of care was altered, including procedure or anesthesia delay, procedure cancellation, and other resource utilization, such as unplanned followup tests or procedures and changes to perioperative patient management. As discussed above in the Statement of Work, rates of other outcomes without a comparator would not provide interpretable data about the true benefits or harms of routine testing.

Data Extraction and Summaries

Data from each study were extracted by one experienced methodologist. The extraction was reviewed and confirmed by at least one other methodologist. Data were extracted into customized forms in the Systematic Review Data Repository at http://srdr.ahrq.gov. Relevant data captured included publication information, study design, intervention and comparator arms, baseline characteristics, outcome definitions, results, and study quality. The forms were tested on several studies and revised before the commencement of full data extraction.

Quality Assessment

We assessed the methodological quality of studies based on predefined criteria. We used a three-category grading system (Low, Medium, or High Risk of Bias) to denote the methodological quality of each study as described in the AHRQ methods guide.[16] This system defines a generic grading scheme that is applicable to varying study designs, including RCTs, nonrandomized comparative trials, and cohort studies. We reviewed the Cochrane Risk of Bias list,[17] the amended Newcastle-Ottawa Scale for cohort studies (http://www.ohri.ca/programs/clinical_epidemiology/oxford.asp), the McMaster Quality Assessment Scale for Harms (McHarms),[18,19] and a list of quality measures commonly used by EPCs for relevant questions. We used all the concepts from the Cochrane Risk of Bias list but chose simpler, more straightforward questions from other sources.

For RCTs, we asked about clarity of eligibility criteria, avoidance of inappropriate exclusions, representativeness of the included patients, adequacy of the patient descriptions, full definitions of outcomes, outcome assessment blinding, dropout rate, use of intention-to-treat analyses, accounting for multicenter studies, reporting clarity without discrepancies, appropriateness of randomization technique, and allocation concealment. We omitted patient and caretaker blinding since this would not be feasible for almost all studies.

For nonrandomized studies, we asked about clarity of eligibility criteria, avoidance of inappropriate exclusions, representativeness of the included patients, adequacy of the patient descriptions, full definitions of outcomes, outcome assessment blinding, dropout rate, accounting for multicenter studies, reporting clarity without discrepancies, selection of the nonexposed cohort, and whether analyses adjusted for any baseline characteristics or confounders.

For cohort studies, we asked about clarity of eligibility criteria, avoidance of inappropriate exclusions, representativeness of the included patients, adequacy of the patient descriptions, full definitions of outcomes, dropout rate, reporting clarity without discrepancies, and whether a consecutive or random sample of patients was enrolled.

Based on the responses to the quality questions, we determined a risk of bias for each study. This was based on an overall assessment of the study. As a general guide, we used the following formulation.

Low Risk of Bias. These studies have the least apparent bias, and their results are considered valid. They generally possess the following: a clear description of the population, setting, interventions, and comparison groups; appropriate measurement of outcomes; appropriate statistical and analytic methods and reporting; no reporting errors; clear reporting of dropouts and a dropout rate less than 20 percent; and no obvious bias.

Medium risk of bias. These studies are susceptible to some bias, but it is not sufficient to invalidate the results. They do not meet all the criteria for low risk of bias due to some deficiencies, but none are likely to introduce major bias. They may be missing information, making it difficult to assess limitations, including risk of bias per se, and potential problems.

High risk of bias. These studies have been judged to carry a significant risk of bias that may invalidate the reported findings. These studies have serious errors in design, analysis, or reporting and contain discrepancies in reporting or have large amounts of missing information.

Data Synthesis

We summarized all included studies in narrative form, as well as in summary tables (see below) that condense the important features of the study populations, design, intervention, outcomes, and results.

For comparisons of the same intervention and control arms in patients scheduled for sufficiently similar surgical procedures with the same outcomes in at least three studies, we performed DerSimonian & Laird random effects model meta-analyses of RRs.[20] For each meta-analysis, the statistical heterogeneity was assessed with the I^2 statistic, which describes the percentage of variation across studies that is due to heterogeneity rather than chance.[21,22]

To provide estimates of summary complication rates from cohort (single-group) studies, we performed simple pooling (dividing the sum of events by the sum of total patients), which is equivalent to a fixed effect model meta-analysis of proportions. This approach was chosen because it was the simplest and best accounted for the heterogeneity across studies and small numbers of events. The purpose of these summary estimates is only to compare reported rates of complications, not to determine a generalizable estimate of complication rates.

Minimal Important Difference

P values, and by extension 95 percent confidence intervals (CI), assess the statistical significance of a difference between interventions (or other comparisons). Of greater relevance for users of the evidence is the concept of clinical significance, which addresses the question of whether a difference is clinically important. With sufficient power, a study can easily find a highly statistically significant difference that is of little importance to a patient, clinician, or other decisionmaker. To address this issue, with input from the TEP, we made a priori definitions for a line of difference in relation to clinically important thresholds, which are referred to as minimally important differences (MID).[23] The MID is a clearly defined clinical threshold, below which the evidence (effect estimates and corresponding CIs) shows no meaningful difference and above which the evidence shows a benefit or harm of one intervention over another.[24] Notably, for the purposes of a comparative effectiveness review, the utility of MID pertains primarily to bodies of evidence for which there is sufficient evidence.

We determined different MIDs for different outcomes. For mortality and major or severe life- or health-altering morbidities and complications (such as stroke, myocardial infarction, or life-threatening hemorrhage), the MID is 0 percent when determining if there is a clinically important difference. For this low risk (and generally low-cost) intervention (preoperative testing), any difference is of concern to patients and clinicians. In other words, all statistically significant differences are deemed to be clinically important. However, to make the determination that there is evidence of no difference, we used a threshold of 20 percent. Thus, only in cases where the 95 percent CI of a difference was within the boundaries of 0.80 to 1.20 (on the relative risk [RR] scale), did we determine that there was evidence of no important difference.

For other, noncritical outcomes, we also used a MID of 20 percent, based on agreement that smaller differences would not be clinically important. To determine that there is evidence of a clinically important difference, the 95 percent CI of the difference had to be fully beyond 0.80 or 1.20 (on the RR scale). Alternatively, to determine that there is evidence of no clinically important difference, the 95 percent CI of the difference had to fully within the range of 0.80 to 1.20 on the RR scale.

Grading the Body of Evidence

We graded the strength of the body of evidence as per the AHRQ methods guide.[16] Based on the division of outcomes within the Key Questions, we determined the strengths of evidence for the following three categories of outcomes: 1) clinical outcomes; 2) intermediate outcomes; and 3) harms.

We summarized study limitations, directness, consistency, precision, publication and reporting bias, and other issues. Study limitations (based on risk of bias) were defined as low, medium, or high based methodological quality, as described above. Directness pertained to whether the studies directly compared the interventions and the relevance of the specific outcomes assessed. We assessed the consistency of the data as either "no inconsistency" or "inconsistency present" (or not applicable, if there was only one study) based on the direction and magnitude of effects across studies. Precision was based primarily on whether the effect estimates fell within the MID. A precise estimate would allow a clinically useful conclusion based on the MID. An imprecise estimate was one for which the CI is wide enough to preclude a conclusion based on the MID. We evaluated publication and outcome reporting bias as a single domain (Reporting Bias) per AHRQ draft methods.[10,24] The domain was assessed only if there was sufficient evidence based on the other four domains.[24] Quantitative methods to assess reporting bias, including funnel plots, were planned if at least 10 studies reported an outcome for a given testing scenario.[24] When there were fewer studies, we assessed the completeness of reporting of each outcome across studies and investigated unexplained statistical heterogeneity to assess the likelihood of reporting bias.[10,24]

We rated the strength of evidence for a particular comparison for each outcome category using one of the following four labels (as per the AHRQ methods guide): high, moderate, low, or insufficient. Ratings were assigned based on our level of confidence that the evidence reflected the true effect for the major comparisons of interest. Ratings were defined as follows:

16

High. We are very confident that the estimate of effect lies close to the true effect for this outcome. The body of evidence has few or no deficiencies. We believe that the findings are stable (i.e., another study would not change the conclusions).

Moderate. We are moderately confident that the estimate of effect lies close to the true effect for this outcome. The body of evidence has some deficiencies. We believe that the findings are likely to be stable, but some doubt remains.

Low. We have limited confidence that the estimate of effect lies close to the true effect for this outcome. The body of evidence has major or numerous deficiencies (or both). We believe that additional evidence is needed before concluding either that the findings are stable or that the estimate of effect is close to the true effect.

Insufficient. We have no evidence, we are unable to estimate an effect, or we have no confidence in the estimate of effect for this outcome. No evidence is available or the body of evidence has unacceptable deficiencies, precluding reaching a conclusion

We further assessed the body of evidence regarding its applicability to the U.S. population of patients undergoing surgical procedures. Where appropriate we assessed whether the studies were applicable to patients undergoing a specific procedures (e.g., cataract surgery) or to patients undergoing a category of procedures (e.g., children having general surgery). The assessment of applicability took into account the range of surgeries investigated, the severity of illness and other features of the included patients, and the currency of the evidence (e.g., whether the studies were done within the past 10 years).

Peer Review

The initial draft report was prereviewed by the TOO and an AHRQ Associate Editor (a senior member of a sister EPC). Following revisions, the draft report was sent to invited peer reviewers and simultaneously uploaded to the AHRQ Web site where it was available for public comment for 30 days. All reviewer comments (both invited and from the public) were collated and individually addressed. The revised report and the EPC's responses to invited and public reviewers' comments were again reviewed by the TOO and Associate Editor prior to completion of the report. The authors of the report had final discretion as to how the report was revised based on the reviewer comments, with oversight by the TOO and Associate Editor.

Results

The literature search yielded 4,581 citations (Appendix A). From these, 220 articles were provisionally accepted for review based on abstracts and titles (Figure 2). After screening the full text, 57 studies (in 58 articles) were found to have met the inclusion criteria. Fourteen of the 57 studies were comparative,[25-39] and the remainder were single-group studies.[4,5,40-81] The Summary Tables, with the descriptions and results of each study, are in Appendix C.

The remaining 160 retrieved articles were rejected for not meeting the eligibility criteria (see Appendix B for the list of rejected articles and the reasons for their rejection). The most common reasons for article rejection were that the article only analyzed test results as predictor of association with outcomes, the test evaluated in the article was not performed on all patients (only ad hoc testing done where testing was done at the clinician's discretion), the article was non-comparative and did not include a process outcome (e.g., surgical delay/cancellation, followup testing), the article was not a primary study, the article dealt with a surgery or procedure that did not involve anesthesia, the test reported was not a test of interest, the diagnostic test study design was not appropriate, the test was performed to diagnose or evaluate severity/stage of illness, or the article could not be retrieved.

The study designs and baseline characteristics of the 57 studies are shown in Appendix C, Table C1-3. They include six RCTs; one prospective, six retrospective, and one combined prospective and retrospective nonrandomized studies; 22 prospective and 21 retrospective cohort (noncomparative, single group) studies. Three RCTs were focused on cataract surgery, two RCTs and six nonrandomized studies focused on general or various surgeries, one RCT focused on vascular surgery, and one nonrandomized comparative study each focused on tonsillectomy and orthopedics. Overall, the studies evaluated the preoperative tests for the following procedures: general or various surgeries (37 studies), tonsillectomy (5 studies), cataract surgery (4 studies), orthopedic surgery (4 studies), vascular surgery (3 studies), head and neck/ear, nose, throat (ENT) surgery (2 studies), and one study each for neurosurgery and electroconvulsive therapy (ECT). Seventeen of the studies were conducted in children, 25 in adults, and 15 in a mixed population of adults and children.

The studies were conducted in the U.S. (30), England (5), Thailand (4), France (4), Canada (4), Italy (3), Brazil (1), Spain (1), India (1), Kuwait (1), Belgium (1), the Ivory Coast (1), and Saudi-Arabia (1). Forty studies were published before 2000, including seven of the 14 comparative studies; 17 studies were published after 2000. Thirteen studies had a high risk of bias, 10 had a medium risk of bias, and 34 had a low risk of bias.

The preoperative tests evaluated in the studies fall into the following categories: basic metabolic panel (electrolytes, kidney function, glucose), extended metabolic panel (liver function tests [LFT] and other serum tests), blood counts (including hemoglobin, hematocrit, white blood cells, and platelets), hemostasis tests (including prothrombin time [PT], partial thromboplastin time [PTT], and bleeding time), urinalysis, pregnancy tests, ECG, chest x ray (CXR), pulmonary function testing (PFT), and echocardiography. The specific tests used in the comparative studies are included in tables within each surgery-specific section of the Results; for cohort studies, see Appendix C Table C-4).

The Results section is structured as follows: the first major section presents the comparative studies (both RCTs and nonrandomized studies), followed by a summary of the cohort studies. Within the comparative study section, the results are divided by category of surgery, within which each Key Question and subquestion is addressed. Within the cohort study section, the results are again divided by category of surgery (or procedure).

Figure 2. Literature flow

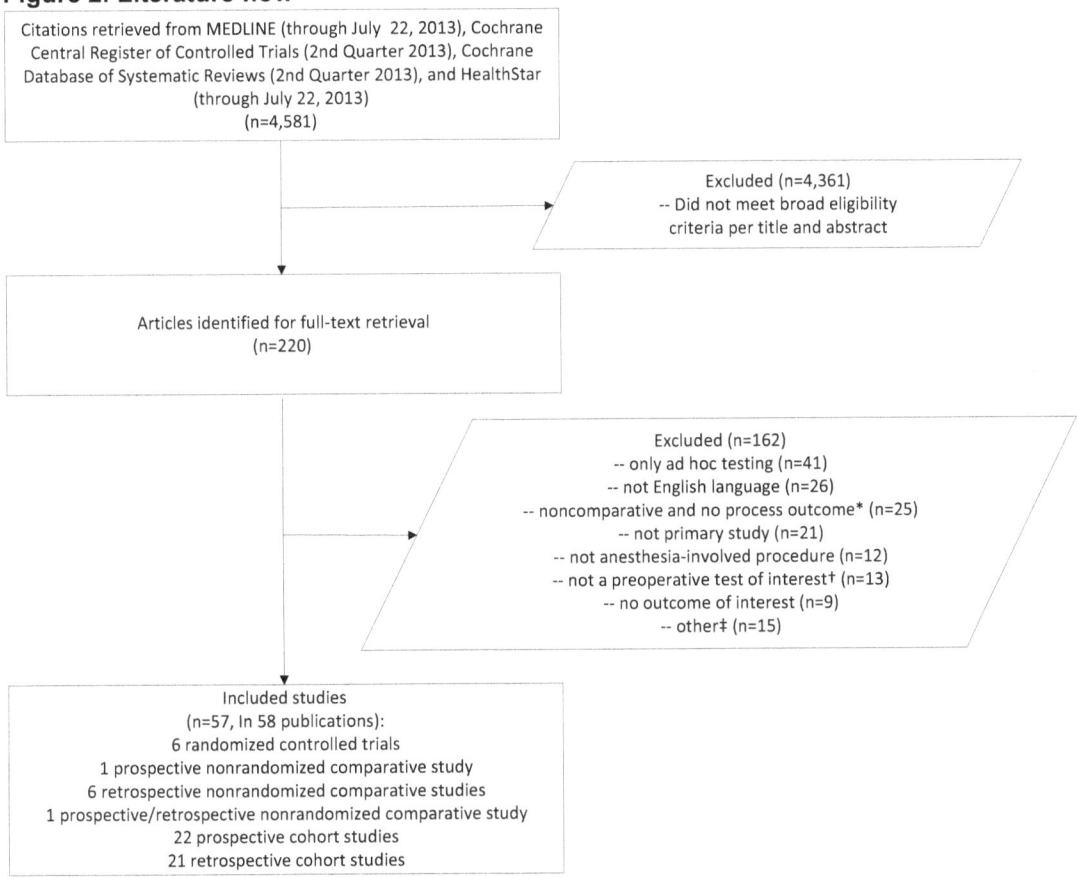

* The "process" outcomes included procedure or anesthesia delay, procedure cancellation, and other resource utilization, including unplanned followup tests or procedures and changes to perioperative patient management.
† Thallium scintigraphy, heart rate variability, Holter monitor, iron status.
‡ Analyses of combined tests and history and physical examination, analysis of only abnormal test results, analysis of test results as predictor of associations with outcomes, case report, could not retrieve article, diagnostic test, emergency surgery or trauma, mix of elective and emergency surgery, no results specific to preoperative tests, not an evaluation of routine preoperative tests, trial of preoperative interventions, referral to preoperative clinic, survey of anesthesiologists, test performed to diagnose or evaluate severity or stage of illness, too unclear a link between test results and subsequent management.

Comparative Studies

Six RCTs (in seven publications)[26,29-31,33,36,37] and one prospective,[27] six retrospective,[25,28,32,34,35,38] and one combined prospective and retrospective nonrandomized study[39] compared alternative strategies regarding the use of routine or per protocol preoperative testing. Three RCTs were focused on cataract surgery, two RCTs and six nonrandomized studies were conducted in adults or children (two studies) undergoing a variety of minor or elective or routine surgeries, one RCT was conducted in adults undergoing vascular surgery, one nonrandomized study was conducted in adults undergoing orthopedic surgery, and one nonrandomized study was conducted in children undergoing tonsillectomy and/or adenoidectomy.

The comparative studies were conducted in the U.S. (six studies), Canada (3 studies), Italy (2 studies), Brazil (1 study), the Ivory Coast (one study), and England (one study). Among the RCTs, four were deemed to have a low risk of bias and two a medium risk of bias (Appendix D Table D-1). Among the nonrandomized studies, all were deemed to have high risk of bias (Appendix D Table D-2).

Cataract Surgery

Three RCTs (in four articles) randomized adults undergoing cataract surgery (Appendix C Tables C-1 and C-2 and Tables 3 and 4).[26,30,31,33] Two of the trials (from the United States and Brazil) had similar eligibility criteria, excluding patients under 40 or 50 years of age, those receiving general anesthesia, or those who had had a recent myocardial infarction. The third (Italian) trial also included only patients undergoing local anesthesia but excluded those undergoing anticoagulant or insulin therapy. All compared routine preoperative testing in all patients with no required testing (ad hoc testing generally allowed if warranted). All have been published since 2000. The Brazilian and Italian studies were deemed to have a low risk of bias. The U.S. study was deemed to have a medium risk of bias, primarily because it was a multicenter study, which was not accounted for in the analyses.

In all three trials, routine testing included an ECG (Table 3). One trial described the remaining tests only as "routine medical tests."[26] The other two trials included a complete blood count. One included glucose, and one included a full basic metabolic panel.

All trials found no significant differences in perioperative complication rates (Appendix C Table C-5). The RRs of various specific perioperative complications ranged from 0.70 to 2.0 (P=0.30-1.00) and all 95% CI spreads were broader than 0.77 (lower CI) to more than 1.34 (upper CI). Only the Schein et al. trial found evidence of no clinically important difference (based on an MID of 0.8-1.2) for total intraoperative and postoperative (up to 1 week) complications; there were 301 complications in each arm, resulting in RR = 1.00 (95% CI 0.85, 1.17). The trials each lumped or split complications differently, but generally reported on intraoperative and postoperative ophthalmic complications and systemic complications including acute anxiety, cardiovascular events, respiratory events, and metabolic events (see Appendix C Table C-5). By meta-analysis (Figure 3), the studies were consistent (homogeneous), and the summary RR = 0.99 (95% CI 0.86, 1.14) indicated overall evidence of no clinically important difference in perioperative complication rates between routine and ad hoc testing. The much larger Schein et al. trial (with 19,000 patients) provided 80 percent of the weight to the meta-analysis, but the smaller studies were fully consistent in their findings with the large trial.

Two of the cataract trials also reported on rates of procedure cancellation.[30,33] The studies had RRs of 1.00 (95% CI 0.42, 2.38) and 0.97 (95% CI 0.78, 1.21), with wide confidence intervals, suggesting no difference in cancellation rates. (Appendix C Table C-6).

No trial reported on quality of life or satisfaction, surgical delay, change in anesthesia or procedure plan, or resource utilization. No trial addressed Key Question 2 regarding harms of routine preoperative testing.

Subgroup Analyses

The studies consistently found no evidence of a difference in outcomes between those who did or did not have routine preoperative tests. Therefore, no differences in outcomes could be discerned among the specific type of anesthesia planned (all excluded general anesthesia), comorbidities, other patient characteristics (in general, all were over 40 or 50 years old), or who ordered the tests (this was generally not reported). These trials compared routine (everyone tested) versus no or ad hoc testing, so there is no evidence specifically regarding per protocol testing. The trials did not provide evidence regarding possible differences in outcomes based on the length of time prior to the procedure that the tests were conducted.

Summary: Cataract Surgery

Three RCTs—two with low, one with moderate risk of bias—compared routine versus no (or ad hoc) preoperative testing with ECG, basic metabolic panel, and CBC for patients undergoing cataract surgery. The studies were clinically similar to each other and consistent; there is a high strength of evidence of no clinically important difference in complication rates. By meta-analysis, for total complications, the RR = 0.99 (95% CI 0.86, 1.14). There is also a high strength of evidence suggesting that routine testing does not affect rates of procedure cancellation, but the confidence intervals were too wide to definitely exclude clinically important (i.e., more than 20 percent) difference. No other outcomes were reported. The evidence is inadequate to evaluate potential differences based on subgroups of patients. Overall, there is no evidence of different outcomes related to routine preoperative testing (Table 4).

Table 3. Comparative study: Tests by study arm in cataract surgery

Author Year PMID	Arm	ECG	CXR	Basic Metabolic	Extended Metabolic	CBC	Hemostasis Tests	Urinalysis	Pregnancy Test	Stress Test	Echo	Other
Cavallini 2004 15506597	Routine	Yes										"Routine medical tests"
	No testing											
Lira 2001 11558245	Routine	Yes		Glucose		Yes						
	No testing*											
Schein 2000 10639542	Routine	Yes		Electrolytes, BUN, creatinine, glucose		Yes		Yes				
	No testing											

BUN = blood urea nitrogen; CBC = complete blood count; CXR = chest x ray; ECG= electrocardiogram; Echo = echocardiogram. * Some undefined testing was allowed if "the patient presented with anew or worsening medical problem that would warrant medical evaluation with testing, even if surgery were not planned."

Table 4. Routine or per protocol versus ad hoc preoperative testing: Strength of evidence domains for cataract surgery

Outcome	Surgery	Tests	Study Design: No. Studies (N)	Study Limitations	Directness	Consistency	Precision	Reporting Bias	Other Issues	Strength of Evidence
Perioperative complications, total	Cataract surgery	ECG, metabolic panel, CBC	RCT: 3 (21,531)	Medium	Direct	Consistent	Precise	Undetected	None	High
Procedure cancellation	Cataract surgery	ECG, metabolic panel, CBC	RCT: 2 (20,562)	Low	Direct	Consistent	Precise	Undetected	None	High

CBC = complete blood count; CI = confidence interval; ECG = electrocardiogram; N/A = not applicable (when strength of evidence is insufficient based on the other four domains); NRS = nonrandomized comparative study; RCT=randomized controlled trial.

Figure 3. Perioperative total complications in cataract surgery: Routine versus ad hoc testing

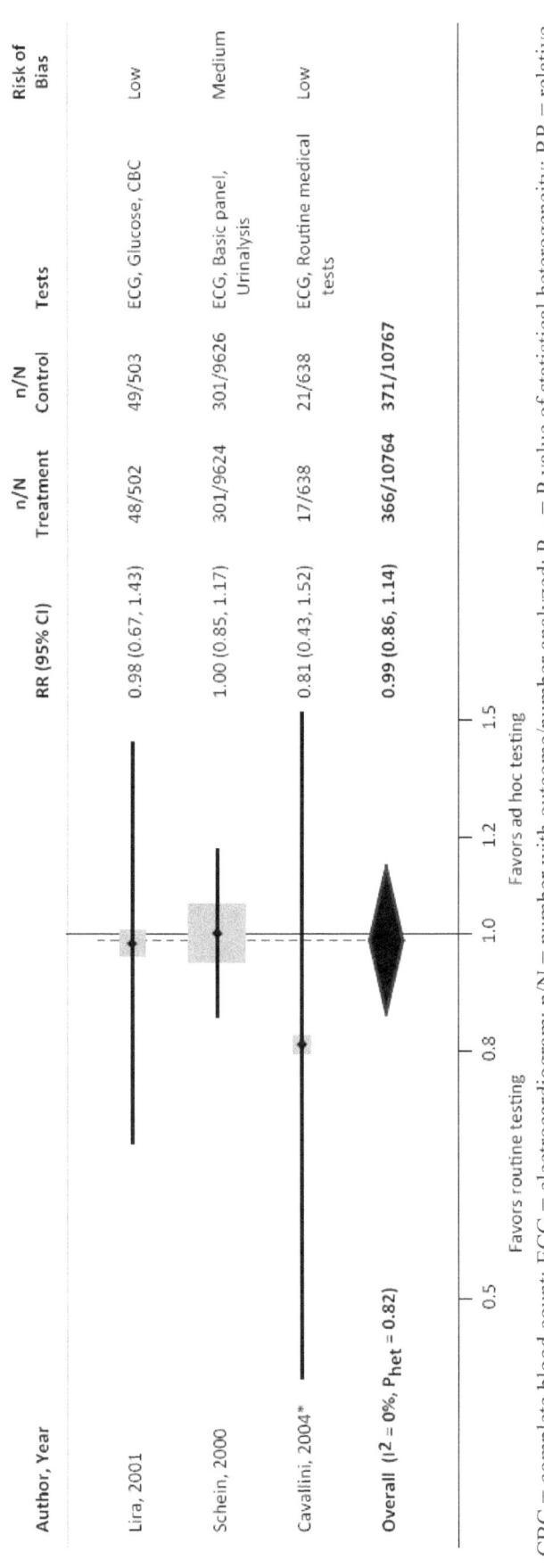

Author, Year	RR (95% CI)	n/N Treatment	n/N Control	Tests	Risk of Bias
Lira, 2001	0.98 (0.67, 1.43)	48/502	49/503	ECG, Glucose, CBC	Low
Schein, 2000	1.00 (0.85, 1.17)	301/9624	301/9626	ECG, Basic panel, Urinalysis	Medium
Cavallini, 2004*	0.81 (0.43, 1.52)	17/638	21/638	ECG, Routine medical tests	Low
Overall ($I^2 = 0\%$, $P_{het} = 0.82$)	0.99 (0.86, 1.14)	366/10764	371/10767		

CBC = complete blood count; ECG = electrocardiogram; n/N = number with outcome/number analyzed; P_{het} = P value of statistical heterogeneity; RR = relative risk.

* Total complications not reported; assumes that all reported complications were independent of each other.

23

General or Various Surgeries, Adults

One RCT [36] and four nonrandomized studies (one prospective [27] and three retrospective[25,28,34]) compared routine or per protocol testing with ad hoc or no testing in adults undergoing a variety of elective surgeries. A sixth nonrandomized study (combined prospective and retrospective) compared routine and per protocol testing [39] (Appendix C Tables C-1, C-2, C-7, Tables 5–7). These studies included general, orthopedic, urologic, neurologic, and other surgeries;[27,36] elective noncardiac surgeries;[25,39] cataract surgery, transurethral resection of the prostate, laparoscopic cholecystectomy, hip arthroplasty, abdominal hysterectomy, breast reduction, radical neck dissection, any cardiovascular surgery, and any thoracic surgery surgeries;[28] and "ambulatory" surgery.[34] The studies generally included all patients who underwent the indicated surgeries, except that the prospective study excluded patients undergoing dialysis.[27] As described in the following paragraphs, each study evaluated a different panel of tests. Two of the retrospective nonrandomized studies were published in 1989 and 1994, the combined prospective and retrospective study was published in 1996; the other studies were published in 2005 and 2009. The nonrandomized studies all have a high risk of bias, primarily because their analyses did not adjust for baseline characteristics or other differences among the compared groups in these three studies, including patient characteristics, surgeries performed, surgeons and anesthesiologists, their experience, or other confounders. Particularly for the three retrospective studies that all compared outcomes for time periods at their hospitals before and after a change in testing policy, the lack of adjustment for covariables and confounders is a substantial analytic flaw that calls into question the validity of their findings. The RCT was rated as having a low risk of bias.

The RCT (Chung et al.[36]) compared per protocol ECG, CXR, basic metabolic panel, CBC, coagulation tests, and sickle cell testing with no testing (except for day-of-surgery glucose for people with diabetes and ad hoc testing was allowed at the discretion of the anesthesiologist) (Table 5).

The prospective nonrandomized study (Finegan et al.[27]) compared routine testing, using ECG, CXR, basic and extended metabolic panels, CBC, hemostasis tests, and urinalysis, with ad hoc use of the same tests at the discretion of the staff anesthesiologist or anesthesiology resident (Table 5), but did not adjust their analyses.

The three retrospective studies compared outcomes for time periods at their hospitals before and after an algorithm, hospital policy, or program defining protocols for preoperative testing was implemented. In no study was testing done routinely in all patients. The per protocol testing in Larocque et al.[28] consisted of ECGs in patients at least 40 years old or with cardiovascular or pulmonary disease, CXRs in patients with cardiovascular or pulmonary disease, basic metabolic panels (or just glucose), extended metabolic panels, and hemostasis tests by indication; all patients had CBCs and urinalysis (Table 5). Importantly, testing was generally more common in the ad hoc group than in the per protocol group and rates of testing with ECG, hemostasis tests, and urinalysis were very similar between groups (Table 5). Almanaseer et al.[25] evaluated the implementation of recommendations for preoperative testing based on the 2002 ACC/AHA guideline update for perioperative cardiovascular evaluation for noncardiac surgery,[82] although details regarding the protocol were not reported. As part of implementing the ACC/AHA recommendations, patients had clinical evaluations but all analyses were based on the use of per protocol testing. Wyatt et al.[34] evaluated a standardized preadmission screening program that included per protocol ECG in patients at least 40 years old; CXR in patients at least 50 years old;

and routine basic and extended metabolic panels, CBC, prothrombin time (PT), and urinalysis in all patients.

The final study (Mignonsin et al.[39]) compared a retrospective period when patients routinely were tested with ECG, CXR, basic metabolic panel, CBC, hemostasis tests, urinalysis and hemoglobin electrophoresis, and a prospective period when patients were tested per a protocol based on H&P. Of note, during the "routine" period many patients did not receive the recommended tests, although usually more patients were tested than during the per protocol period. The percentages who were tested during the routine and per protocol periods were: ECG 67 and 47 percent, CXR 71 and 37 percent, glucose 92 and 38 percent, creatinine 45 and 15 percent, blood urea nitrogen 90 and 9 percent, CBC 95 and 59 percent, partial thromboplastin time 35 and 0 percent, urinalysis 58 and 0.5 percent. However, prothrombin time and hemoglobin electrophoresis were less commonly conducted during the routine period (50% and 12%) than during the per protocol period (99.5% and 27%). The patients underwent elective surgeries, including gastrointestinal, trauma/orthopedic, urologic, and gynecologic. The study may have been conducted in the Ivory Coast (the location of the surgeries was unclear).

Perioperative complications were reported in five of the studies (Table 6, Appendix C Table C-7). The RCT, Chung et al., "intraoperative events" occurred at the same rate in both patients with per protocol and no testing (1.4%; RR = 1.0; 95% CI 0.4, 3.0). Almanaseer et al. reported results only for specific perioperative complications; they did not report total complications. Using a Poisson model to allow for multiple events per person, there was a borderline nonsignificant difference favoring per protocol testing (21/314; 6.7%) over ad hoc testing (31/261; 12%) with RR = 0.56 (95% CI 0.31, 1.01).

Among the specific complications reported, only pneumonia occurred significantly more commonly among the ad hoc than the per protocol testing group. Other complications reported included myocardial infarction, heart failure, unstable angina, cardiac death, stroke, renal failure, pneumonia, respiratory failure, and noncardiac death (Appendix C Table C-7). Finegan et al. reported significantly more total perioperative complications in patients with ad hoc than per protocol testing (by Chi squared or Fisher's exact tests; ad hoc: 16 complications in 8/431 [1.9%] patients vs. per protocol: 4 complications in 4/507 [0.8%] patients; RR = 0.43 [95% CI 0.13, 1.40]). The study also found significantly more deaths and episodes of renal failure in the ad hoc cohort (4/431 [0.9%] vs. 0/507 for both death and renal failure). Other complications were not reported per study arm; overall, complications included heart failure (3 patients), myocardial infarction (2 patients), deep vein thrombosis (2 patients), stroke (1 patient), and pneumonia (1 patient). Larocque et al. also reported significantly more total complications in patients undergoing ad hoc testing (13%) than per protocol testing (9.2%) They reported a P value of <0.001 by Chi squared or Fisher's exact tests, but our calculation of the RR was nonsignificant (RR=0.73; 95% CI 0.51, 1.04). The study failed to find that any specific perioperative complication was more common with ad hoc testing only. A long list of complications were reported, including specific infectious, cardiac, respiratory surgical trauma, gastrointestinal, genitourinary, neurologic, and miscellaneous complications (Appendix C Table C-7). The study evaluated deaths and complications based on whether they may have been attributable to any preoperative tests, either done or not done. They concluded that neither of the deaths and none of the complications were attributable to any specific test.

The studies lumped many tests ordered for patients undergoing many different types of surgeries. It is reasonable to assume that there are undetected differences in effects based on which tests were used and which surgeries people underwent. Due to the clinical differences across studies in patients, surgeries, and testing protocols, we did not meta-analyze the results from these studies.

Among the specific perioperative complications, in-hospital death was reported by four of the studies (Table 6, Appendix C Table C-7). All studies reported lower perioperative death rates in the groups undergoing routine (or per protocol) testing. The same caveats about interpretation of the complications results apply to the death results. Notably, there were few deaths in all studies.

Larocque et al. also reported nonsignificantly higher rates of return to the operating room and of prolonged hospital stay (not defined) for patients who had ad hoc (both outcomes: 4/492, 0.8%) rather than per protocol testing (both outcomes: 1/501, 0.2%; RR = 0.25; 95% CI 0.03, 2.19) (Appendix C Tables C-8 & C-10). Similarly, Almanaseer et al. found that patients who underwent ad hoc testing had almost statistically significantly longer hospital lengths of stay (mean 6.5, range 1-42 days) compared to those who had testing per protocol (mean 5.6, range 1-30 days; P = 0.055) (Appendix C Table C-11).

For all reported outcomes, there was no clear difference in effect between Larocque et al.,[28] published in 1994, and the more recent studies published in 2005. However, given advances in surgical management over the past 20 years, the applicability of the older studies may be limited.

Only Wyatt et al., which was published in 1989, reported on surgical cancellation. Including miscellaneous and unknown reasons for cancellation, the rates of cancellation were similar with ad hoc (127/1834, 6.9%) and per protocol testing (261/4058, 6.4%; RR = 0.93; 95% CI 0.76, 1.14) (Appendix C Table C-6). The study also reported numbers of patients who had their surgeries canceled because of specific tests; however, the study failed to report the numbers of patients who had each of the tests, hampering the ability to analyze these data. Significantly more cancellations occurred due to laboratory tests. Of note, though, is the fact that three of the four cancellations (across both study arms) due to abnormal CXRs were in patients with known pulmonary disease and all nine cancellations due to abnormal ECGs were in patients with known cardiac disease.

Almanaseer et al. found no significant difference in the proportion of patients who had their surgery deferred (delayed) before or after the testing algorithm was implemented (3.3% vs. 4.7%, respectively; RR = 1.33; 95% CI 0.61, 2.88) (Appendix C Table C-12).

No trial reported on quality of life or satisfaction, change in anesthesia or procedure plan, or resource utilization. No trial addressed Key Question 2 regarding harms of routine preoperative testing.

Subgroup Analyses

The studies did not report outcomes specific to any subgroups of interest and did not differ appreciably from each other based on any of the subgroup characteristics. Therefore, no differences in outcomes could be discerned among the specific type of anesthesia planned, comorbidities, other patient characteristics, who ordered the tests (this was generally not reported), or whether testing was conducted per protocol or routinely. The trials did not provide evidence regarding possible differences in outcomes based on the length of time prior to the procedure that the tests were conducted.

Summary: General or Various Surgeries, Adults

One low risk of bias RCT and four high risk of bias nonrandomized studies compared routine (2 studies) or per protocol testing (3 studies) with ad hoc testing, using ECG, CXR, basic and extended metabolic panels, CBC, hemostasis tests, and urinalysis in adult patients undergoing a broad range of elective surgeries. A sixth study compared time periods when patients were to receive either routine testing (during a retrospective period) or per protocol testing (during a prospective period) with a large number of tests. None of the nonrandomized studies adjusted for baseline differences in patient characteristics, types of surgery, surgeons or anesthesiologist, their experience, or other confounders. They also did not analyze how or whether the routine or per protocol tests were linked to resulting outcomes (complications). The RCT reported only on complications, of which there were only a small number; therefore, this trial was underpowered to provide any reliable estimate of relative differences in complications. We have no confidence in the estimate of effects across these studies due to these methodological deficiencies, the important clinical heterogeneity (differences) across all studies, and the high risk of bias of the nonrandomized studies (particularly related to lack of necessary adjustments). Another point that may call into question the validity of the four studies that evaluated ad hoc testing [25,27,28,34] is that the single study to report testing rates in the ad hoc group (Larocque et al.[28]) had similar or higher rates of testing than the per protocol group. This decrease in testing was the goal of implementing the protocol. Thus, comparisons with ad hoc testing do not adequately assess the actual effect of routine or per protocol testing, since the comparator is not no testing.

There is insufficient evidence regarding perioperative complications (Table 7). There is also insufficient evidence of a clinically significant difference in the rate of perioperative death. The clinical heterogeneity of studies, without reporting of subgroup analyses of patients or procedures within studies, further precludes a conclusion about which patients would benefit from routine testing. There is also insufficient evidence regarding other specific outcomes, including return to the operating room, prolonged hospital stay, or surgical cancellation or delay. No trial reported on quality of life or satisfaction, change in anesthesia or procedure plan, or resource utilization. A single high risk of bias nonrandomized study provided insufficient evidence regarding the comparison of routine and per protocol testing. Given the deficiencies in the evidence across studies, it was not possible to compare the effects of routine and per protocol testing. No trial addressed Key Question 2 regarding harms of routine preoperative testing. The evidence is inadequate to evaluate potential differences based on subgroups of interest.

Table 5. Comparative study: Tests by study arm in general/various surgeries in adults

Author Year PMID	Arm	ECG	CXR	Basic Metabolic	Extended Metabolic	CBC	Hemostasis Tests	Urinalysis	Pregnancy Test	Stress Test	Echo	Other
Almanaser 2005 15528897	Per protocol	ACC/AHA Class I*								ACC/AHA Class I*	ACC/AHA Class I*	2002 ACC/AHA cardiac workup, Coronary angiography; ACC/AHA Class I*
	Ad hoc	Yes									ACC/AHA Class I*	
Chung 2009 19151274	Per protocol	>45 yo, cardiac history or HTN	Pulmonary disease or "heavy" smoker	Electrolytes, creatinine if taking diuretics, renal disease, or DM; Glucose if diabetes		>60 yo or suspected anemia	PT, PTT If on anticoagulant, coagulopathy, or chronic liver disease					Sickle cell if African or Caribbean origin
	No testing			Glucose of diabetes (on day of surgery)								

28

Table 5. Comparative study: Tests by study arm in general/various surgeries in adults (continued)

Author Year PMID	Arm	ECG	CXR	Basic Metabolic	Extended Metabolic	CBC	Hemostasis Tests	Urinalysis	Pregnancy Test	Stress Test	Echo	Other
Finegan 2005 15983141	Routine	Yes	Yes	Electrolytes, creatinine, BUN, glucose	ALP, bilirubin	Yes	PT-INR, PTT	Yes				
	Ad hoc	Yes	Yes	Electrolytes, creatinine, BUN, glucose	ALP, bilirubin	Yes	PT-INR, PTT	Yes				
Larocque 1994 7922901	Per protocol	77% of patients †	45% of patients †	Electrolytes (76% of patients), Glucose (65% of patients)†	LFTs (6% of patients)	Yes	INR, PTT (23% of patients)†	93% of patients				
	Ad hoc	75% of patients	57% of patients	Electrolytes (97% of patients), Glucose (95% of patients)	LFTs (11% of patients)	Yes	INR, PTT (26% of patients)	97% of patients				
Mignonsi, 1996 8762245	Routine	67% of patients	71% of patients	Glucose (92% of patients), Creatinine (45% of patients), Urea (90% of patients)		95% of patients	PT (50% of patients); PTT (35% of patients)	58% of patients				Hb electrophoresis (12% of patients)

29

Table 5. Comparative study: Tests by study arm in general/various surgeries in adults (continued)

Author Year PMID	Arm	ECG	CXR	Basic Metabolic	Extended Metabolic	CBC	Hemostasis Tests	Urinalysis	Pregnancy Test	Stress Test	Echo	Other
	Per protocol	47% of patients	37% of patients	Glucose (38% of patients), Creatinine (15% of patients), Urea (9% of patients)		59% of patients	PT (100% of patients); PTT (0% of patients)	0.5% of patients				Hb electrophoresis (27% of patients)
Wyatt 1989 2729769	Per protocol	≥40 yo	≥50 yo	Na, K, glucose, BUN, creatinine, CO_2, Cl	LFTs, Ca, P, uric acid, cholesterol	Yes	PT, PTT	Yes				
	Ad hoc	Yes	Yes	Na, K, glucose, BUN, creatinine, CO_2, Cl	LFTs, Ca, P, uric acid, cholesterol	Yes	PT, PTT					EtOH, Cardiac enzymes

ALP = alkaline phosphatase; BUN = blood urea nitrogen; Ca = calcium; CBC = complete blood count; Cl = chloride; CO_2 = carbon dioxide; CXR = chest x ray; ECG = electrocardiogram; Echo = echocardiogram; EtOH = alcohol; HTN = hypertension; K = potassium; LFT = liver function tests; Na = sodium; P = phosphorus; PT-INR = prothrombin time and international normalized ratio; PTT = partial thromboplastin time; yo = years old

* American College of Cardiology/American Heart Association Class I recommendations: ECG: If recent chest pain or ischemic equivalent in clinically intermediate- or high-risk patients scheduled for an intermediate- or high-risk operative procedure; Stress test: If intermediate pretest probability of CAD, significant change in clinical CAD status; Echo: Left ventricular function, resting (if current or poorly controlled heart failure); Coronary angiography: if high risk of adverse outcome based on noninvasive tests, angina unresponsive to adequate medical therapy, unstable angina, equivocal noninvasive tests in patients at high clinical risk undergoing high-risk surgery

† ECG: ≥40 yo, cardiovascular disease, pulmonary disease; CXR: cardiovascular disease, pulmonary disease; Electrolytes: >70 yo, diabetes mellitus, renal disease, taking corticosteroids digitalis diuretic; Glucose: diabetes mellitus, taking corticosteroids; INR, PTT: bleeding disorder, hepatobiliary disease, malignancy, vascular disease, taking anticoagulants

Table 6. Perioperative complications of general or various surgeries

Author Year PMID	Study Design Risk of Bias	Tests	Outcome	Arm	N Analyzed	Events (%)	RR (95% CI)
Almanaseer 2005 15528897	rNRS High	ECG, Cardiac tests per ACC/AHA guideline	Total complications*	Per protocol testing / Ad hoc testing	314 / 261	21 (6.7%) / 31 (11.9%)	0.56 (0.33, 0.96)
			Death, total	Per protocol testing / Ad hoc testing	314 / 261	1 (0.3%) / 3 (1.1%)	0.28 (0.03, 2.65)
			Pneumonia	Per protocol testing / Ad hoc testing	314 / 261	2 (0.6%) / 8 (3.1%)	0.21 (0.04, 0.97)
			Renal failure	Per protocol testing / Ad hoc testing	314 / 261	4 (1.3%) / 3 (1.1%)	1.11 (0.25, 4.91)
Chung 2009 19151274	RCT Low	ECG, CXR, Basic panel, CBC, Hemostasis tests, Sickle cell	Total complications (nonspecified)	Per protocol / No testing	527 / 499	7 (1.3%) / 7 (1.4%)	0.95 (0.33, 2.68)
			Postoperative morbidity	Per protocol / No testing	527 / 499	21 (4.0%) / 16 (3.2%)	1.24 (0.66, 2.35)
			Arrhythmia	Per protocol / No testing	527 / 499	2 (0.4%) / 2 (0.4%)	0.95 (0.13, 6.7)
			HTN	Per protocol / No testing	527 / 499	2 (0.4%) / 2 (0.4%)	0.95 (0.13, 6.7)
			Hypotension	Per protocol / No testing	527 / 499	1 (0.2%) / 0 (0%)	Not calculated
			Oxygen desaturation	Per protocol / No testing	527 / 499	2 (0.4%) / 0 (0%)	Not calculated
			Laryngospasm	Per protocol / No testing	527 / 499	0 (0%) / 2 (0.4%)	Not calculated
			Bronchospasm	Per protocol / No testing	527 / 499	0 (0%) / 1 (0.2%)	Not calculated
			Nausea	Per protocol / No testing	527 / 499	3 (0.6%) / 4 (0.8%)	0.71 (0.16, 3.16)
Finegan 2005 15983141	pNRS High	ECG, CXR, Basic panel, CBC, Extended panel, Hemostasis tests, Urinalysis	Perioperative surgical Complications	Routine testing / Ad hoc testing	507 / 431	4 (0.8%) / 8 (1.9%)	0.43 (0.13, 1.40)
			Death	Routine testing / Ad hoc testing	507 / 431	0 (0%) / 4 (0.9%)	Not calculated
			Renal failure	Routine testing / Ad hoc testing	507 / 431	0 (0%) / 4 (0.9%)	Not calculated

31

Table 6. Perioperative complications of general or various surgeries (continued)

Author Year PMID	Study Design Risk of Bias	Tests	Outcome	Arm	N Analyzed	Events (%)	RR (95% CI)
Larocque 1994 7922901	NRS High	ECG, CXR, Basic panel, Extended panel, CBC, Hemostasis tests, Urinalysis	Perioperative surgical	Per protocol testing	501	46 (9.2%)	0.71 (0.49, 1.01)
			Complications	Ad hoc testing	492	64 (13%)	
			Morbidity attributable to test†	Per protocol testing	501	0 (0%)	Not calculated
				Ad hoc testing	492	0 (0%)	
			Death	Per protocol testing	501	0 (0%)	Not calculated
				Ad hoc testing	492	2 (0.4%)	
			Death, attributable to test†	Per protocol testing	501	0 (0%)	Not calculated
				Ad hoc testing	492	0 (0%)	
			Pneumonia	Per protocol testing	501	0 (0%)	Not calculated
				Ad hoc testing	492	7 (1.4%)	
Mignonsin, 1996 8762245	p,rNRS High	ECG, CXR, Basic panel, CBC, Hemostasis test, Urinalysis, Hb Electrophoresis	Bleeding	Routine	200	1 (1%)	Not calculated
				Per protocol	200	0 (0%)	
			Delayed awakening	Routine	200	0 (0%)	Not calculated
				Per protocol	200	1 (0.5%)	
			Death	Routine	200	0 (0%)	Not calculated
				Per protocol	200	0 (0%)	
			Postoperative morbidity	Routine	200	0 (0%)	Not calculated
				Per protocol	200	0 (0%)	

ACC/AHA = American College of Cardiology/American Heart Association; CBC = complete blood count; CI = confidence interval; CXR = chest x ray; ECG = electrocardiogram; pNRS = prospective nonrandomized (comparative) study; p =rNRS = combined pro- and retrospective nonrandomized (comparative) study; p =rNRS = retrospective nonrandomized (comparative) study; RR = relative risk

* Assuming that each patient who had a complication had only one of the reported complications (i.e., that the complications were independent of each other).
† Attributable to preoperative laboratory investigation(s), either done or not done

Table 7. Routine or per protocol testing: Strength of evidence domains for general/various surgeries in adults

Outcome	Surgery	Tests	Study Design: No. Studies (N)	Study Limitations	Directness	Consistency	Precision	Reporting Bias	Other Issues	Strength of Evidence
Routine or per protocol vs. ad hoc testing										
Perioperative complications, total	Various, adults	Multiple*	NRS: 5 (3932)	High	Direct	Consistent	Imprecise†	Undetected	Unadjusted analyses	Insufficient
Perioperative death	Various, adults	Multiple*	NRS: 4 (2906)	High	Direct	Consistent	Imprecise†	Undetected	Unadjusted analyses	Insufficient
Perioperative complications, specific (selected)	Various, adults	Multiple*	NRS: 3 (2506)	High	Direct	NA	Variable	N/A	Unadjusted analyses	Insufficient
Return to operating room	Various, adults	Multiple*	NRS: 1 (993)	High	Direct	NA	Imprecise	N/A	Unadjusted analysis	Insufficient
Procedure cancellation	Various, adults	Multiple*	NRS: 1 (5892)	High	Direct	NA	Precise	N/A	Unadjusted analysis	Insufficient
Procedure delay	Various, adults	Multiple*	NRS: 1 (575)	High	Direct	NA	Imprecise	N/A	Unadjusted analysis	Insufficient
Length of stay	Various, adults	Multiple*	NRS: 1 (575)	High	Direct	NA	Imprecise	N/A	Unadjusted analysis	Insufficient
Routine vs. per protocol testing										
Perioperative complications, total	Various, adults	Multiple	NRS: 1 (575)	High	Direct	NA	Imprecise	N/A	Unadjusted analysis	Insufficient
Perioperative death	Various, adults	Multiple	NRS: 1 (575)	High	Direct	NA	Imprecise	N/A	Unadjusted analysis	Insufficient
Perioperative complications, specific (selected)	Various, adults	Multiple	NRS: 1 (575)	High	Direct	NA	Imprecise	N/A	Unadjusted analysis	Insufficient

CBC = complete blood count; CI = confidence interval; ECG = electrocardiogram; N/A = not applicable (when strength of evidence is insufficient based on the other four domains); NRS = nonrandomized comparative study; RCT = randomized controlled trial. * ECG, CXR, basic and extended metabolic panels, CBC, coagulation tests, and urinalysis
† Summary RR 95% does not meet 20% threshold for MID

33

Orthopedic Surgery, Adults

A single retrospective nonrandomized study, published in 1999,[38] evaluated preoperative testing in adults (including children >16 years old) undergoing various elective orthopedic (foot/ankle, knee, hand/wrist, shoulder) surgeries (Appendix C Tables C-1, C-2). The study compared routine testing with ECG, CXR, CBC, basic and extended metabolic profiles, urinalysis, hemostasis tests, and syphilis testing with per protocol use of CBC for all and ECG for patients greater than 45 years old (Table 8). It was deemed to be of high risk of bias, primarily because of the retrospective study design without appropriate adjustments and inadequate reporting of the analysis. Only one relevant outcome was reported, unplanned hospital admission or readmission within 30 days of surgery (Table 9, Appendix C Table C-9). There was no significant difference in unplanned hospital admission or readmission within 30 days of surgery between the two groups (P>0.6).

No other relevant outcomes were reported. No subgroup analyses were reported.

Summary: Orthopedic Surgery, Adults

There is insufficient evidence regarding the comparison of routine versus per protocol preoperative testing in adults undergoing orthopedic surgery (Table 9). A single high-risk-of bias retrospective nonrandomized study found no difference in the rate of unplanned hospital admissions within 30 days of surgery.

Table 8. Comparative study: Tests by study arm in orthopedic surgery

Author Year PMID	Arm	ECG	CXR	Basic Metabolic	Extended Metabolic	CBC	Hemostasis tests	Urinalysis	Pregnancy Test	Stress Test	Echo	Other
Mancuso 1999 10203622	Routine	Yes	Yes	Yes	Yes	Yes	PT, PTT, ESR	Yes				RPR
	Per protocol	≥50 yo				Yes						

CBC = complete blood count; CXR = chest x ray; ECG = electrocardiogram; Echo = echocardiogram; ESR = erythrocyte sedimentation rate; PT = prothrombin time; PTT = partial thromboplastin time; RPR = reactive plasma regain.

Table 9. Routine or per protocol versus ad hoc preoperative testing: Strength of evidence domains for orthopedic surgery

Outcome	Surgery	Study Design: No. Studies (N)	Tests	Study Limitations	Directness	Consistency	Precision	Reporting Bias	Other Issues	Strength of Evidence
Unplanned hospital admission	Orthopedics, Adults	NRS: 1 (640)	Various	High	Direct	NA	Imprecise	N/A	Unadjusted analyses	Insufficient

CI = confidence interval; N/A = not applicable (when strength of evidence is insufficient based on the other four domains); NRS = nonrandomized comparative study.

35

Vascular Surgeries, Adults

One low risk of bias RCT,[37] published in 2003, compared routine stress dobutamine echocardiography versus no testing in people undergoing vascular surgery (Table 10). Three outcomes were reported, perioperative cardiac death, respiratory death, and congestive heart failure or elevated troponin I levels. (Table 11, Appendix C Table C-13). The trial was small, with only 99 patients, and there were few perioperative complications, including no cardiac deaths and only a single respiratory death in a patient who did not have a preoperative stress echocardiogram. A perioperative cardiac event occurred in 3/53 (5.7%) of patients without testing and 1/46 (2.2%) of patients with testing, yielding a RR = 0.38 (95% CI 0.04, 3.57).

No other relevant outcomes were reported. No subgroup analyses were reported.

Summary: Vascular Surgery, Adults

There is insufficient evidence regarding the comparison of routine versus per protocol preoperative testing in adults undergoing vascular surgery (Table 11). A single low risk of bias RCT failed to find differences in rates of perioperative death or cardiac complications.

Table 10. Comparative study: Tests by study arm in vascular surgery

Author Year PMID	Arm	ECG	CXR	Basic Metabolic	Extended Metabolic	CBC	Hemostasis tests	Urinalysis	Pregnancy Test	Stress Test	Echo	Other
Falcone 2003 14689407	Routine										Yes	
	No testing											

CBC = complete blood count; CXR = chest x ray; ECG = electrocardiogram; Echo = echocardiogram; ESR = erythrocyte sedimentation rate; PT = prothrombin time; PTT = partial thromboplastin time; RPR = reactive plasma regain.

Table 11 Routine preoperative testing: Strength of evidence domains for vascular surgery

Outcome	Surgery	Tests	Study Design: No. Studies (N)	Study Limitations	Directness	Consistency	Precision	Reporting Bias	Other Issues	Strength of Evidence
Cardiac death	Vascular	Echo	RCT: 1 (99)	Low	Direct	NA	Imprecise	N/A		Insufficient
Respiratory death	Vascular	Echo	RCT: 1 (99)	Low	Direct	NA	Imprecise	N/A		Insufficient
Cardiac complication	Vascular	Echo	RCT: 1 (99)	Low	Direct	NA	Imprecise	N/A		Insufficient

CI = confidence interval; Echo = dobutamine stress echocardiogram; N/A = not applicable (when strength of evidence is insufficient based on the other four domains); NRS = nonrandomized comparative study.

General or Various Surgeries, Children

One English RCT [29] and an Italian nonrandomized study [32] evaluated preoperative testing in children undergoing various elective surgeries (Appendix C Tables C-1, C-2, Tables 12 and 13).

The RCT[29] (which was published in 1975) compared a routine basic metabolic panel, an extended metabolic panel, and hemoglobin with routine hemoglobin only in all pediatric surgical patients expected to stay in the hospital less than 1 week (Table 12). It was deemed to be of medium risk of bias, primarily because inadequate reporting of the study design hampered assessment of their methods. The study did not report which specific surgeries were included. The only reported pertinent outcome was hospital length of stay (Appendix C Table C-11). There was no significant difference in length of stay between the two group (P>0.1). Those children who had the full panel of tests performed routinely had a mean hospital stay of 3.7 days (no range or measure of variability was reported); those who had only the routine hemoglobin performed had a mean hospital stay of 3.4 days.

The retrospective nonrandomized study,[32] published in 1998, included children (who had not been delivered preterm) with ASA physical status 1 or 2 who underwent "elective minor surgery." The study was deemed to be of high risk of bias, primarily because it failed to adjust for differences between the groups. The study compared an earlier 3-year period when it was hospital policy to routinely perform hemoglobin, urinalysis, creatine phosphokinase, and cholinesterase with a later 12-year period when there was no policy regarding preoperative testing (Table 12). The results of the study are unadjusted, but they reported that the two study groups were comparable with respect to age, type of surgery, and ASA physical status classification. Major complications occurred rarely (2/1884 [0.11%] during routine testing; 4/8772 [0.05%] during ad hoc testing) with RR = 2.33 (95% CI 0.43, 12.7). Minor complications were more common, but all resolved without sequelae (routine 292/1884 [15%] vs. ad hoc 1123/8772 [13%]); although the rates were similar (15% vs. 13%), they were significantly different (RR = 1.21; 95% CI 1.08, 1.36), favoring ad hoc testing. The rates of specific minor complications were also generally more common during the period of routine preoperative testing (Appendix C Table C-7), with clinically important differences for persistent vomiting and restlessness. The study found no significant difference in rates of longer than expected hospital stay because of surgical complications (routine 51/1884 [2.7%] vs. 266/8772 [3.0%]; RR = 0.89; 95% CI 0.66, 1.20) (Appendix C Table C-10). No planned surgeries were canceled due to abnormal test results.

The two studies did not report on other outcomes, including quality of life, satisfaction, surgical delay, change in anesthesia or procedure plan, resource utilization, or harms of routine testing.

Subgroup Analyses

The studies did not provide results data to allow analyses of any differences by subgroups of interest or based on who ordered the tests or the length of time prior to the procedure that the tests were conducted.

Summary: General or Various Surgeries, Children

One RCT from 1975 with medium risk of bias reported limited outcome data. A second retrospective, high risk of bias nonrandomized study failed to provide sufficient evidence regarding the effect on patient and resource outcomes of routine or per protocol preoperative testing. The limited data suggest no difference in length of hospital stay related to routine testing with basic and extended metabolic panels, and a counterintuitive increase in minor perioperative complications with routine preoperative testing. The age of the studies (38 and 15 years) further calls into question the applicability of their findings to modern pediatric surgical management. No study reported on quality of life, satisfaction, surgical delay, change in anesthesia or procedure plan, resource utilization, or harms of routine testing. The evidence is inadequate to evaluate potential differences based on subgroups of interest (Table 13).

Table 12. Comparative study: Tests by study arm in general/various surgeries in children

Author Year PMID	Arm	ECG	CXR	Basic Metabolic	Extended Metabolic	CBC	Hemostasis tests	Urinalysis	Pregnancy Test	Stress Test	Echo	Other
Leonard 1975 1095116	Routine			Na, K, CO_2, BUN, "Reducing sugar"	Ca, P, ALP, total protein, Alb, cholesterol, SGOT, Mg	Hb						
	Routine (Hb only)					Hb						
Meneghini 1998 9483592	Routine					Hb		Yes				CPK, cholinesterase
	No testing											

Alb = albumin; ALP = alkaline phosphatase; BUN = blood urea nitrogen; Ca = calcium; CBC = complete blood count; CO_2 = carbon dioxide; CPK = creatine phosphokinase; CXR = chest x ray; ECG = electrocardiogram; Echo = echocardiogram; Hb = hemoglobin; K = potassium; Na = sodium; Mg = magnesium; P = phosphorus; SGOT = serum glutamic-oxaloacetic transaminase; yo = years old.

Table 13. Routine or per protocol versus ad hoc preoperative testing: Strength of evidence domains for general/various surgeries in children

Outcome	Surgery	Tests	Study Design: No. Studies (N)	Study Limitations	Directness	Consistency	Precision	Reporting Bias	Other Issues	Strength of Evidence
Perioperative complications, total	Various, children	Multiple*	NRS: 1 (10,656)	High	Direct	NA	Imprecise†	N/A	Unadjusted analysis	Insufficient
Perioperative complications, major (total)	Various, children	Multiple*	NRS: 1 (10,656)	High	Direct	NA	Imprecise†	N/A	Unadjusted analysis	Insufficient
Perioperative complications, specific (selected)	Various, children	Multiple*	NRS: 1 (10,656)	High	Direct	NA	Variable	N/A	Unadjusted analyses	Insufficient
Procedure cancellation	Various, children	Multiple*	NRS: 1 (10,656)	High	Direct	NA	Imprecise	N/A	Unadjusted analysis	Insufficient
Length of stay	Various, children	Multiple*	RCT: 1 (789) NRS: 1 (10,656)	High	Direct	Consistent	Imprecise	N/A	Unadjusted analyses	Insufficient

CBC = complete blood count; CI = confidence interval; ECG = electrocardiogram; N/A = not applicable (when strength of evidence is insufficient based on the other four domains); NRS = nonrandomized comparative study; RCT=randomized controlled trial.

* Nonrandomized study evaluated hemoglobin, urinalysis, creatine phosphokinase, and cholinesterase

† Summary RR 95% does not meet 20% threshold for MID

Tonsillectomy and/or Adenoidectomy, Children

A single retrospective nonrandomized study, published in 1997, compared perioperative complication rates among children scheduled for tonsillectomy and/or adenoidectomy (Appendix C Tables C-1, C-2, Tables 14 and 15).[35] Zwack et al. compared the patients of 11 surgeons who routinely tested all patients with the hemostasis tests PT and partial thromboplastin time (PTT) and the patients of two surgeons who tested them with PT, PTT, and bleeding time based on their H&P (or if genetic family history information was unavailable) (Table 14). This study was deemed to have a high risk of bias. Of note, the two surgeons who did per protocol testing performed 50 percent more surgeries than the other 11 surgeons combined. The 11 surgeons conducting routine testing (who performed relatively few tonsillectomies) had significantly more perioperative bleeding complications (22/1750 [1.3%]) than the two more experienced surgeons conducting per protocol testing (16/2624 [0.7%]; P=0.027) (Appendix C Table C-14). Only 1 of the 22 children with bleeding complications after routine testing had a minimally abnormal PT (0.1 second above normal). Of the 16 children with bleeding complications after per protocol testing, 8 had normal hemostasis tests and 8 had had no hemostasis testing done.

No other relevant outcomes were reported. No subgroup analyses were reported.

Summary: Tonsillectomy and/or Adenoidectomy, Children

There is insufficient evidence regarding routine (or per protocol) preoperative testing in children undergoing tonsillectomy and/or adenoidectomy (Table 15). A single, flawed, 16 year old, retrospective nonrandomized study found significantly higher rates of perioperative bleeding among patients of less experienced surgeons who routinely conducting hemostasis tests than more experienced surgeons who performed per protocol testing. However, none of the bleeding episodes were related to clinically significant abnormal coagulation tests, and the difference in bleeding rates was more likely to have been related to the experience and surgical volume of the surgeons.

Table 14. Comparative study: Tests by study arm in tonsillectomy

Author Year PMID	Arm	ECG	CXR	Basic Metabolic	Extended Metabolic	CBC	Hemostasis tests	Urinalysis	Pregnancy Test	Stress Test	Echo	Other
Zwack 1997 9051441	Routine					Yes	PT, PTT					
	Per protocol					Yes	PT, PTT, bleeding time (if the history and physical exam were suggestive or genetic [family] information was unavailable)					

CBC = complete blood count; CXR = chest x ray; ECG = electrocardiogram; Echo = echocardiogram; PT = prothrombin time; PTT = partial thromboplastin time.

Table 15. Routine or per protocol vs. ad hoc preoperative testing: Strength of evidence domains for tonsillectomy

Outcome	Surgery	Tests	Study Design: No. Studies (N)	Study Limitations	Directness	Consistency	Precision	Reporting Bias	Other Issues	Strength of Evidence
Perioperative complications, specific (selected)	Tonsillectomy, children	Coagulation tests	NRS: 1 (4374)	High	Direct	NA	Imprecise	N/A	Unadjusted analyses	Insufficient

CBC = complete blood count; CI = confidence interval; ECG = electrocardiogram; N/A = not applicable (when strength of evidence is insufficient based on the other four domains); NRS = nonrandomized comparative study; RCT=randomized controlled trial.

42

Cohort Study Findings

Given how few comparative studies were available, we looked at cohort studies to test the indirect link between testing and outcomes, since if tests can be shown not to affect management, they cannot affect outcomes. The weaknesses with this approach are that it is not possible to determine if the change in management led to better or worse outcomes and that the implicit comparison can be made only with no testing. No implicit comparison can be made with ad hoc testing based on H&P since there are no data on management changes based on the ad hoc testing. For the purposes of this section, we combined data from the true cohort studies and the routine or per protocol arms from the comparative studies. This section focuses on the rates of specific outcomes, and the data from the comparative studies are equivalent to those from the cohort studies. Among the 57 studies eligible for this review, the 47 with relevant outcomes are summarized in this section.

The 47 studies report a total of five "process" outcomes of interest, including change in patient management (4 studies conducted in adults), change in surgical technique (3 studies conducted in adults; 1 study conducted in children), change in anesthetic management (10 studies conducted in adults; 6 studies conducted in children), procedure cancellation (19 studies conducted in adults; 11 studies conducted in children), and procedure or anesthetic delay (19 studies conducted in adults; 7 studies conducted in children). Thirty-three (70%) of the studies were published before 2000. Thirty-nine (83%) of the studies evaluated routine preoperative testing; the other eight evaluated per protocol testing. An important caveat for the analysis of these studies is that, in general, it is only implied that procedure changes or cancellations were truly due to abnormal test results as opposed to changes that may have occurred for reasons separate from testing. While this caveat also applies to the comparative studies, in these analyses there is no reference group for comparison.

We summarize the information extracted from these studies in a series of tables (Appendix C Tables C15-18) and graphs (Figures 4–7). The underlying data, together with additional extracted information, is accessible online (at http://srdr.ahrq.gov/) in the project "Routine Preoperative Testing—Comparative Effectiveness Review 2013".

The tables include information regarding the number of studies reported for each outcome by preoperative test category, the total number of subjects, and the range of patients with a given outcome across studies as a percentage. For each outcome within a preoperative test category, we also provide the combined (summary) percentages by test, along with their 95% confidence intervals. These were calculated by simple pooling (equivalent to fixed effect model for meta-analysis) and thus should not be construed as estimates of the true rates of the outcomes in the broader population. Instead, they provide a simple comparison of the rates found in existing studies across different procedures and tests. The scatter plots present the study specific proportion of subjects with each outcome by procedure. Given the vast clinical heterogeneity across studies, in terms of procedures, populations, and tests ordered, the scatter plots provide only a basic comparison across studies and not a true estimate of rates.

An analysis of all cohort data across outcomes, by publication year, raises a concern regarding the applicability and interpretation of the studies in regard to assessing the degree to which routine or per protocol tests result in changes in patient management. Namely, across all studies, almost all of the most frequent management changes (changes in anesthesia or surgery technique, delays, and cancellations) occurred in studies published prior to 2000. Except for a 5.1 percent rate of procedure delays in one study from 2005,[25] all patient management changes that occurred in over 2 percent of patients were in older studies. As noted, only 8 (17%) studies used per protocol testing. Given the large clinical heterogeneity across studies, of which routine versus per protocol testing was only one difference, it was not possible to distinguish any differences in outcome rates based on whether testing was done routinely or per protocol.

Change in Surgical Technique

Change in surgical technique was reported in three studies conducted in adults,[52,73,79] and one study conducted in children.[76] All studies were published prior to 1998. Three studies evaluated either hemostasis tests, a combined panel with various tests, or CXR in patients undergoing various or general surgical procedures; one study evaluated the outcome of a stress test before vascular surgery. The proportion of patients for whom the surgical technique was changed following the preoperative test was relatively low, ranging between 0 and 0.7 percent (Appendix C Tables C-15, C-23; Figure 4).

Change in Anesthetic Management

Change in anesthetic management was evaluated in 10 studies of adults undergoing various/general procedures[5,41,44,48,52,53,57,61,73,77] and 6 studies conducted in children.[42,43,65,66,75,76] These 16 studies evaluated various preoperative tests, including a metabolic panel (2 adult studies), CXR (4 adult studies and 1 pediatric study), ECG (1 adult study), CBC (1 adult study and 2 pediatric studies), hemostasis (2 adult studies), combined panel with various tests (5 adults studies and 1 pediatric study), pregnancy test (2 pediatric studies).

The proportion of pediatric patients experiencing a change in anesthetic management across all tests is low, ranging between 0 and 2.3 percent. The proportion of adults for whom anesthetic management was changed following any preoperative test or combination of tests was higher, ranging between 0 and 10 percent. The highest proportion (10%) was in the study that evaluated electrolytes as part of the metabolic panel for 1001 patients. Notably, the studies that evaluated combined panels had inconsistent results, with four studies reporting 0 percent of patients experiencing the outcome and one study reporting 9 percent of patients experiencing the outcome (Appendix C Tables C-16, C-19; Figure 5). Among studies published between 1977 and 1988, between 0 and 10.5 percent (median 2.9%) of patients had anesthesia management changed, compared with 0 to 3.7 percent (median 0.1%) in the 1990s and 0 percent from 2002 to 2006. Among studies of routine testing, between 0 and 2.3 percent (median 0%) of patients had anesthesia management changed, compared with 0 to 10.5 percent (median 4.3%) with per protocol testing.

Procedure Cancellation

Procedure cancellation was evaluated in 23 studies conducted in adults [4,5,30,33,34,40,41,47,50,52-54,56-58,61-63,68,69,72,79] and 11 studies conducted in children [32,42,43,49,55,59,65,67,70,71,74,80] (Appendix C Tables C-17, C-20, Figure 6).

The adult studies were conducted in patients undergoing various/general procedures (19 studies), ECT (5), cataract surgery (2), and one of each of the following procedures: head & neck, neurosurgery, orthopedic, and vascular surgery. These studies evaluated variety of preoperative tests. The only test that was evaluated in more than one or two studies was the combined panel test, which was evaluated in 11 studies, but the panel was not consistent across studies. The proportion of patients with procedure cancellation was low, ranging between 0 and 6.4 percent with eight combinations of test and procedure yielding a 0 percent cancellation rate.

The pediatric studies were conducted in children undergoing various/general procedures (6 studies), tonsillectomy (5), and head & neck/ENT surgery (1). The studies evaluated a variety of preoperative tests, including CBC, combined panel (1 study included a panel of the following tests: CBC, CXR, ECG, and metabolic panel; 11 studies included various tests; 1 study included a panel of the following tests: ECG, CXR, basic metabolic, CBC, urinalysis, and pregnancy test; and 1 study included a panel of the following tests: ECG, CXR, basic metabolic, CBC, and HIV), pregnancy test, hemostasis, and sickle cell. The proportion of children with procedure cancellation was relatively low, ranging between 0% - 0.5%.

Among studies published between 1983 and 1989, between 0 and 6.4 percent (median 0.1%) of patients had anesthesia management changed, compared with 0 to 2.0 percent (median 0%) in the 1990s and 0 to 2.0 (median 0%) percent from 2002 to 2009. Among studies of routine testing between 0 and 2.0 percent (median 0%) of patients had anesthesia management changed, compared with 0 to 6.4 percent (median 0.4%) with per protocol testing.

Procedure or Anesthesia Delay

Procedure or anesthetic delay was evaluated in 19 studies conducted in adults [4,5,40,41,44,50,51,54,57,58,62,64,68,69,73,78,79,81] and 7 studies conducted in children [42,59,60,66,71,75,76,80] (Appendix C Tables C-18, C-21, Figure 7).

The adult studies were conducted in patients undergoing various or general surgeries (15 studies) with a variety of tests: seven of the 15 studies evaluated various combined panels, two studies evaluated patients undergoing orthopedic surgery, two studies vascular surgery, one study neurosurgery, and one head & neck/ENT surgery. The proportion of patients with procedure cancellation was relatively small across all procedures and tests, ranging from 0 to 5.1 percent.

The eight studies that evaluated this outcome in pediatric patients included children undergoing various/general procedures (6 studies) with various preoperative tests, including CXR (1 study), CBC (2), urinalysis (1), and pregnancy test (2). The other two studies evaluated the outcome of procedure or anesthetic delay in children undergoing head & neck/ENT surgery with CBC (1) and in children undergoing orthopedic surgery with a combined panel. The proportion of children with procedure or anesthetic delay ranged from 0 to 2.7 percent.

Among studies published between 1977 and 1989, between 0 and 1.2 percent (median 0.5%) of patients had anesthesia management changed, compared with 0 to 3.6 percent (median 0.5%) in the 1990s, and 0 to 5.1 percent (median 0.6%) from 2001 to 2013. Among studies of routine testing between 0 and 3.6 percent (median 0.4%) of patients had anesthesia management changed, compared with 1.0 to 5.1 percent (median 1.1%) with per protocol testing.

Figure 4. Scatter: Change in surgical technique

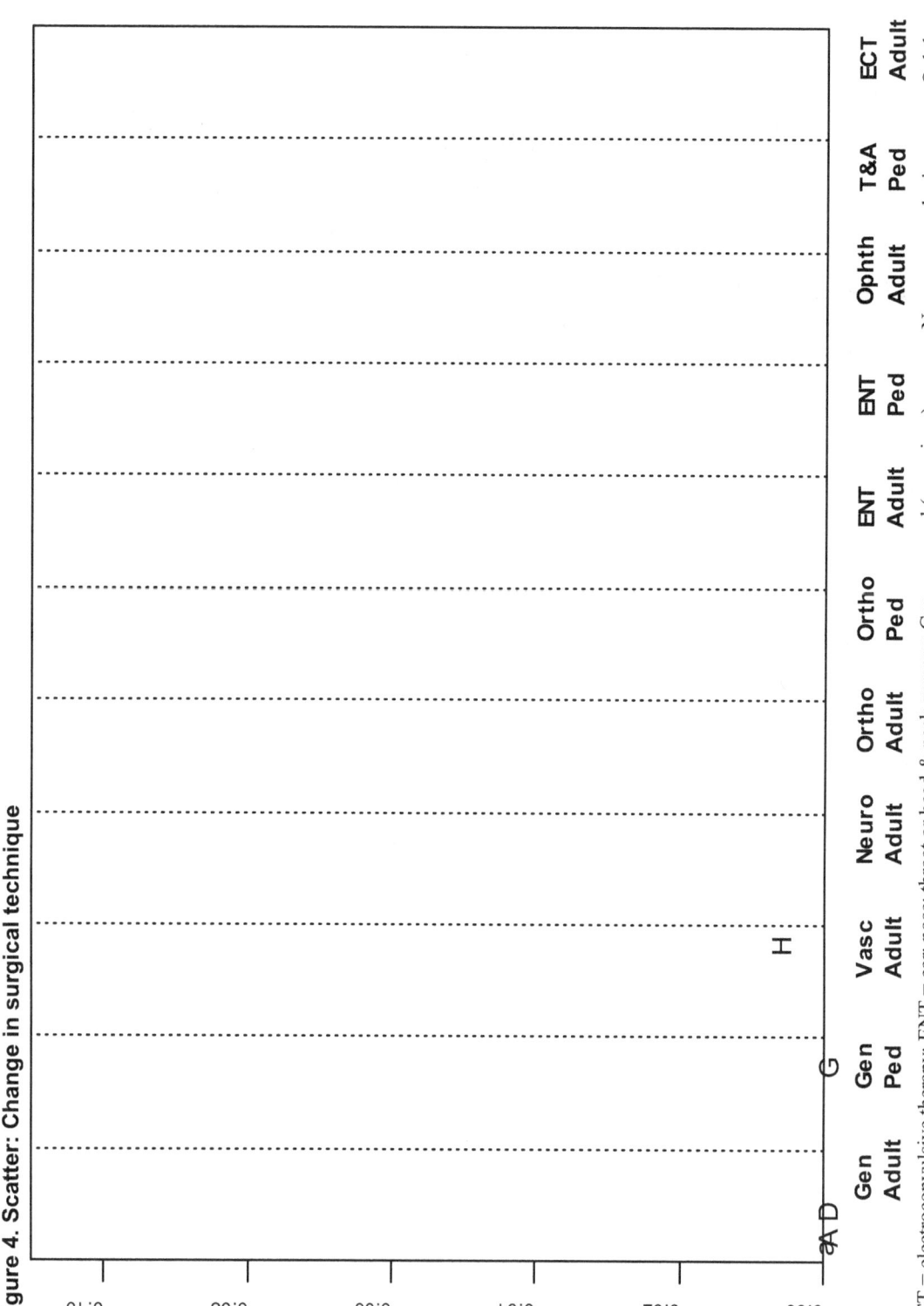

ECT = electroconvulsive therapy; ENT = ear; nose; throat or head & neck surgery; Gen = general (or various) surgery; Neuro = neurologic surgery; Ophth = ophthalmic surgery (including cataract); Ortho = orthopedic surgery; T&A = tonsillectomy and/or adenoidectomy; Vasc = vascular surgery.

a/A = panel of tests; b/B = metabolic tests; c/C = blood counts; d/D = coagulation tests; e/E = urinalysis; f/F = electrocardiogram; g/G = chest x-ray; h/H = cardiac stress test; i/I = pregnancy test; j/J = sickle cell test. Upper case letters indicate routine tests; lower case letters indicate per protocol tests.

Figure 5. Scatter: Change in anesthesia management

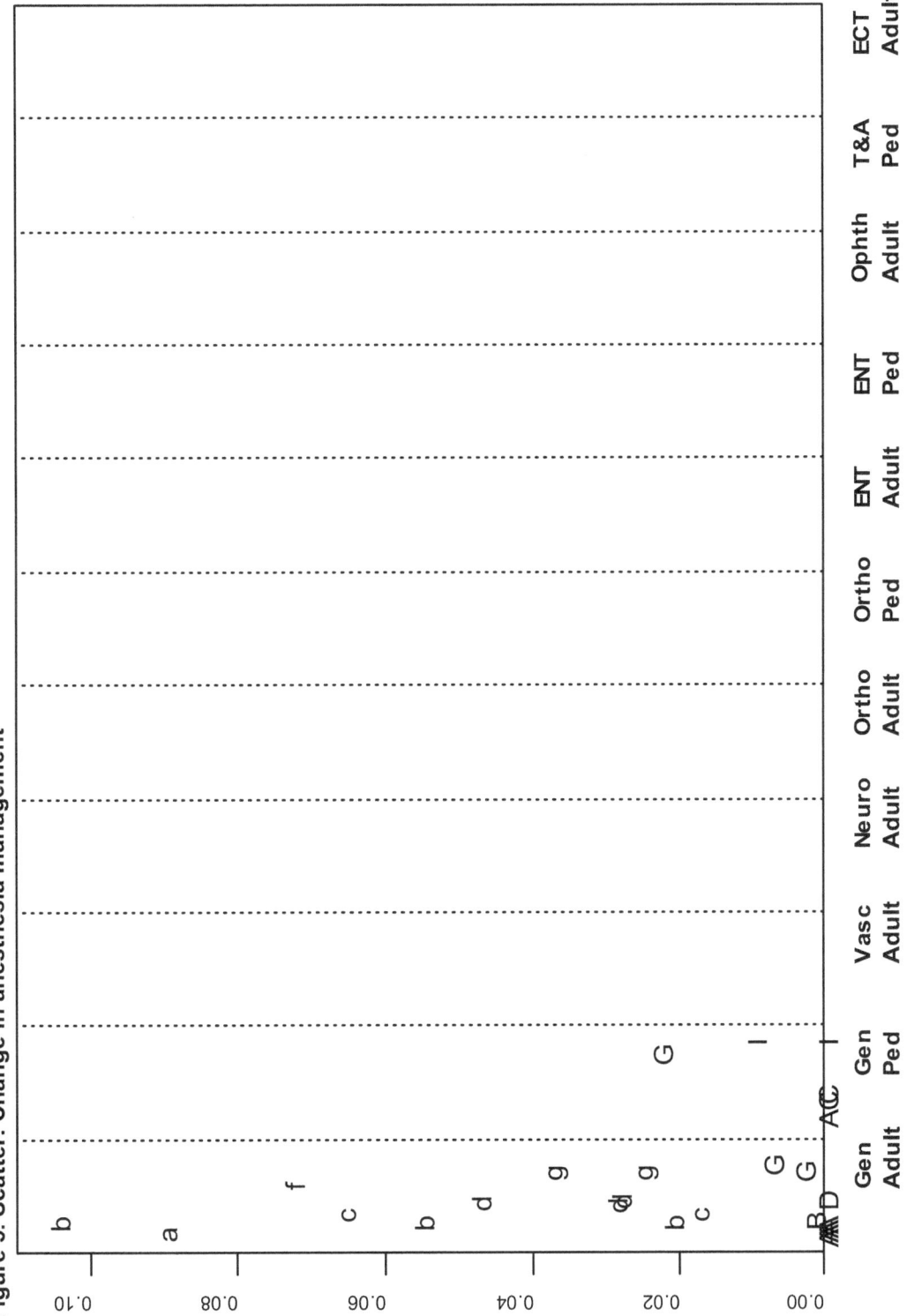

ECT = electroconvulsive therapy; ENT = ear; nose; throat or head & neck surgery; Gen = general (or various) surgery; Neuro = neurologic surgery; Ophth = ophthalmic surgery (including cataract); Ortho = orthopedic surgery; T&A = tonsillectomy and/or adenoidectomy; Vasc = vascular surgery.

a/A = panel of tests; b/B = metabolic tests; c/C = blood counts; d/D = coagulation tests; e/E = urinalysis; f/F = electrocardiogram; g/G = chest x ray; h/H = cardiac stress test; i/I = pregnancy test; j/J = sickle cell test. Upper case letters indicate routine tests; lower case letters indicate per protocol tests.

Figure 6. Scatter: Procedure cancellation

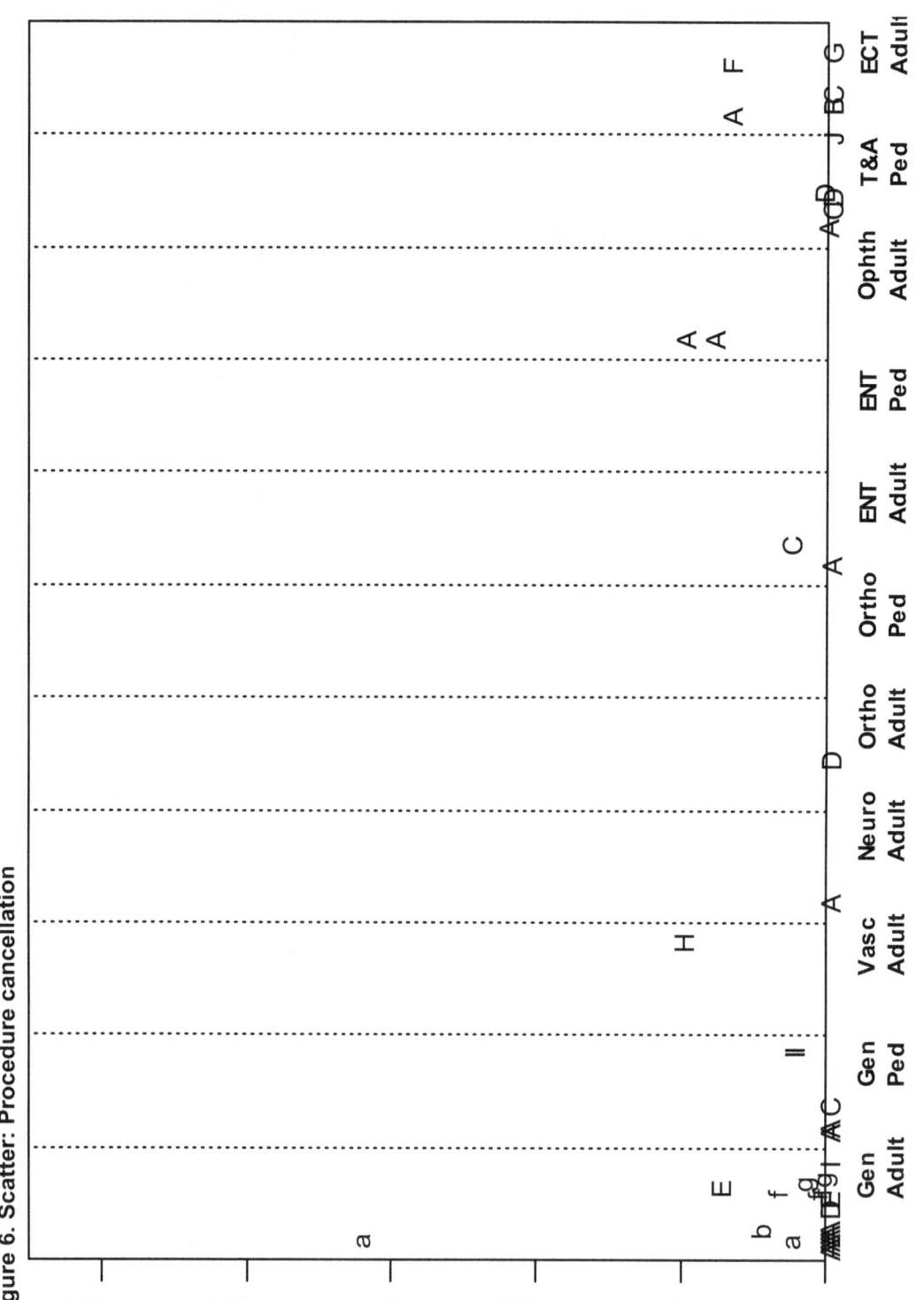

ECT = electroconvulsive therapy; ENT = ear; nose; throat or head & neck surgery; Gen = general (or various) surgery; Neuro = neurologic surgery; Ophth = ophthalmic surgery (including cataract); Ortho = orthopedic surgery; T&A = tonsillectomy and/or adenoidectomy; Vasc = vascular surgery.
a/A = panel of tests; b/B = metabolic tests; c/C = blood counts; d/D = coagulation tests; e/E = urinalysis; f/F = electrocardiogram; g/G = chest x ray; h/H = cardiac stress test; i/I = pregnancy test; j/J = sickle cell test. Upper case letters indicate routine tests; lower case letters indicate per protocol tests.

48

Figure 7. Scatter: Procedure delay

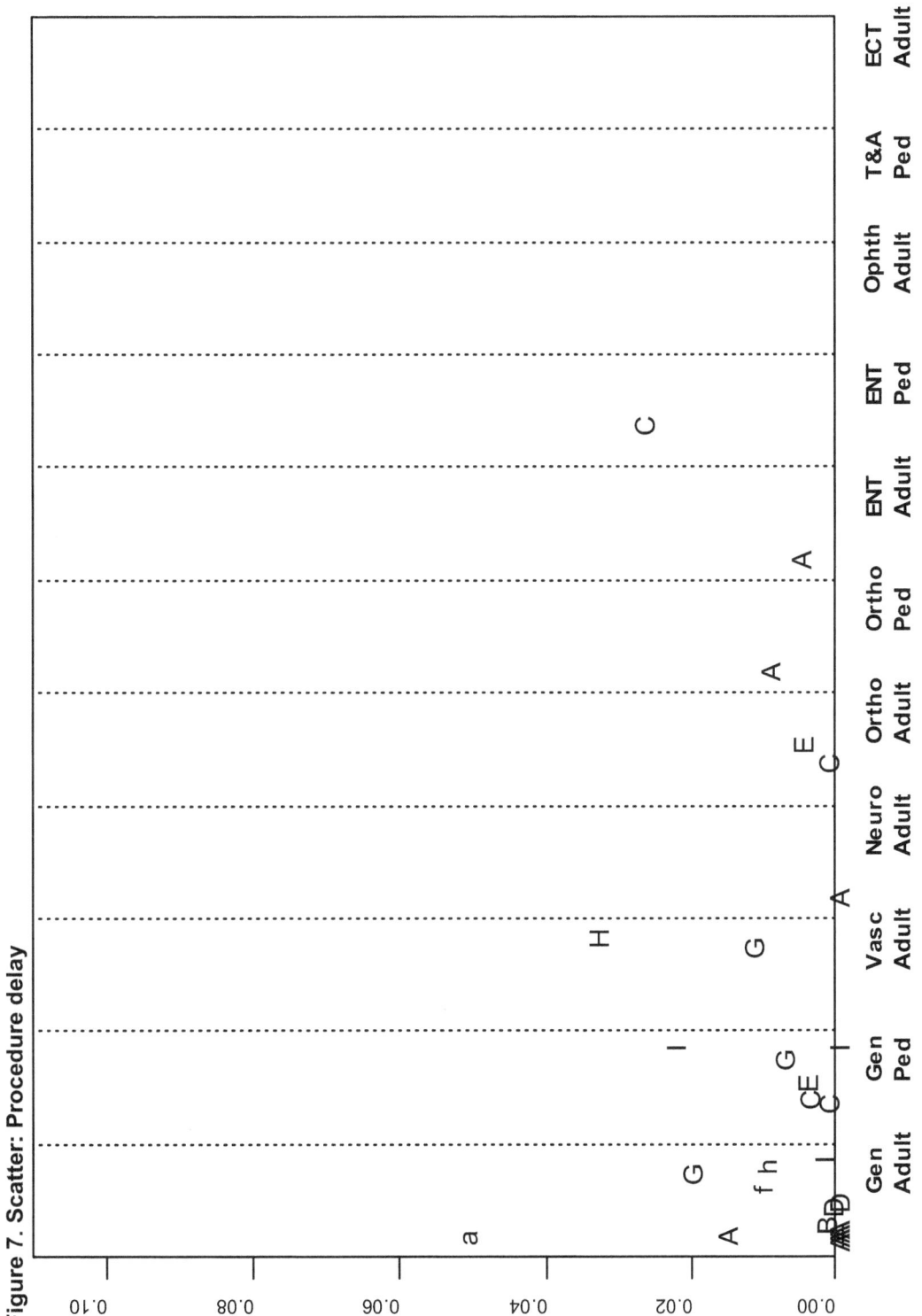

ECT = electroconvulsive therapy; ENT = ear, nose, throat or head & neck surgery; Gen = general (or various) surgery; Neuro = neurologic surgery; Ophth = ophthalmic surgery (including cataract); Ortho = orthopedic surgery; T&A = tonsillectomy and/or adenoidectomy; Vasc = vascular surgery.

a/A = panel of tests; b/B = metabolic tests; c/C = blood counts; d/D = coagulation tests; e/E = urinalysis; f/F = electrocardiogram; g/G = chest x ray; h/H = cardiac stress test; i/I = pregnancy test; j/J = sickle cell test. Upper case letters indicate routine tests; lower case letters indicate per protocol tests.

49

Procedures for Which Testing Did Not Affect Outcomes

As noted, knowing the percentage of patients who had changes in their management provides very limited information regarding whether the tests affects patient outcomes in the absence of a contemporaneous comparison group. It remains unknown whether the patients benefited or were harmed by the changes in management. However, when a study finds that a test (or tests) led to no changes in management, it may be possible to conclude that the test did not affect patient clinical outcomes (other than possibly providing reassurance). However, this conclusion relies on the accuracy of the point estimate (of 0%) and ignores the possibility that the lack of events occurred by random chance. Nevertheless, the following is a summary of the studies and tests that led to no changes in patient management.

Of the 47 studies, 20 reported that the routine or per protocol tests evaluated did not lead to either procedure delay (7 studies),[4,5,40,41,68,69,71] cancellation (17 studies),[4,5,32,40,41,43,47,50,55,58,61-63,65,68-70] change in anesthesia management (5 studies),[5,41,43,61,65] or surgical technique (2 studies).[73,76] No study reported all four outcomes, and only two studies reported three of the outcomes (not change in surgical technique).[5,41]

However, in no scenario (specific test(s) used prior to the same category of procedures in the same population [adults vs. children]) were there at least two studies that both found no changes in patient management.

Nevertheless, among these 20 studies, patients undergoing ECT had no change in management based on CBC, metabolic panel, or CXR (1 study). Adults scheduled for a variety of elective surgeries had no changes in management based on metabolic panels, CBC, hemostasis tests, ECG, urinalysis, or pregnancy test (in 9 of 25 such studies). Children scheduled for a variety of elective surgeries had no changes in management based on metabolic panels, CBC, urinalysis, creatine phosphokinase, cholinesterase, or CXR (in 5 of 10 such studies). In one study each, adults having a panel of tests for neurosurgery, a panel for head & neck surgery, or hemostasis tests for orthopedic surgery had no changes in management. In two (of 5 such studies), children scheduled for tonsillectomy or adenoidectomy had no changes in management based on hemostasis tests, hemoglobin, or sickle cell testing.

Change in Patient Management (With Subgroup Analyses)

Change in patient management was reported in four studies evaluating CBC, CXR, or ECG in adult patients undergoing various/general procedures.[44-46,77] The proportion of patients experiencing this outcome was higher than for any other outcome, ranging between 2.5%-9.9%.

This was not a "clean" outcome for the purposes of this review, since it included medical consultations, new drugs administered, or "further evaluation." However, we included this outcome because it was the only outcome that was analyzed by patient subgroup (Table 16). Four studies evaluated the proportion of various different patient age groups undergoing various/general procedures for the preoperative test of CXR (2 studies), CBC (1 study), or ECG (1 study).

Changes in patient management were reported by age in all studies. In both studies of CXR, change in patient management was significantly or substantially more common in older cohorts (9% among those >60 years old vs. 1-5% in younger cohorts). In two studies, CBC and ECG may have led to changes in management somewhat less frequently in younger people. In two studies that evaluated patients by sex, change in patient management related to ECG occurred equally among men and women, but CXRs yielded significantly more changes in management among men. In one study, the effect of ECG testing on change in patient management was similar among patients with normal and abnormal physical examinations. In another study, CXR resulted in significantly more changes in patient management among patients with a higher ASA category, those with respiratory disease, and those with "major" surgeries planned (as opposed to "minor" or "standard" surgeries), particularly patients undergoing thoracic, cardiac, and vascular surgeries. In summary, these cohort studies confirm a greater impact on management by increasing age, ASA category, and surgery risk.

Summary

In all preoperative testing scenarios for which more than a single study was available (i.e., approaching a sufficient evidence base to form a conclusion) testing resulted in some changes in management. In other words, the evidence suggests that in most situations, routine preoperative testing will result in some delay or cancellation of the procedure (in most studies <2%) or some changes to anesthetic management (up to 11%) or surgical procedure (<1%). However, it is not possible to say whether the changes led to benefit or harm for patients because without a comparator group one cannot assess how the changes in management may have been associated with perioperative outcomes. Two studies suggest that change in management from CXR is more common for older patients (primarily >60 years), and one study each suggests that the effect of ECG is similar in men and women, but that CXR results in change in management in more men, those in a higher ASA risk category, those with respiratory disease, and those with "major" surgeries planned (as opposed to "minor" or "standard" surgeries), particularly patients undergoing thoracic, cardiac, and vascular surgeries. Two studies suggest that change in management from CXR is more common for older patients (primarily >60 years). Two other studies also looked at CXR and ECG by sex and other factors. One of these studies suggests that the effect of ECG is similar in men and women but the second study suggests that CXR results in change in management in more men, those with higher ASA category, those with respiratory disease, and those with "major" surgeries planned (as opposed to "minor" or "standard" surgeries), particularly in patients undergoing thoracic, cardiac, and vascular surgeries. The studies were too clinically heterogeneous to ascertain whether there were any patterns suggesting a difference in process outcomes based on whether preoperative testing was conducted routinely or per protocol.

Table 16. Subgroup analysis of changes in patient management

Author Year PMID	Study Design	Arm	Test	Subgroup	Subgroup Category	N Analyzed	Events (%)	P-value Between Subgroups
Age								
Bhuripanyo 1990 2345323	Retrospective cohort	Routine	CXR	Age	15-29	223	2 (1%)	NR
					30-44	291	3 (1%)	
					45-59	223	12 (5%)	
					≥60	196	17 (9%)	
Bhuripanyo 1995 7622976	Prospective cohort	Routine	CBC	Age	15-29	5	3 (60%)	NR
					30-44	10	8 (80%)	
					45-59	13	11 (95%)	
					≥60	10	8 (80%)	
Bhuripanyo 1992 1293256	Prospective cohort	Routine	ECG	Age	40-49	92	1 (1%)	NR
					50-59	123	4 (3%)	
					60-69	102	3 (3%)	
					≥70	76	2 (3%)	
Silvestri 1999 10713868	Prospective cohort	Per protocol	CXR	Age	≤60	3257	66 (2%)	<0.01
					>60	2636	232 (9%)	
Sex								
Bhuripanyo 1992 1293256	Prospective cohort	Routine	ECG	Sex	Male	145	4 (3%)	NR
					Female	250	6 (2%)	
Silvestri 1999 10713868	Prospective cohort	Per protocol	CXR	Sex	Male	2760	188 (7%)	<0.01
					Female	3306	125 (4%)	
Normal vs. Abnormal physical examination (PE)								
Bhuripanyo 1992 1293256	Prospective cohort	Routine	ECG	PE result	Normal	357	8 (2%)	NR
					Abnormal	38	2 (5%)	
ASA category								
Silvestri 1999 10713868	Prospective cohort	Per protocol	CXR	ASA	ASA 1-2	5062	155 (3%)	<0.01
					ASA 3-5	1018	158 (16%)	

Table 16. Subgroup analysis of changes in patient management (continued)

Author Year PMID	Study Design	Arm	Test	Subgroup	Subgroup Category	N Analyzed	Events (%)	P-value Between Subgroups
Coexisting diseases								
Silvestri 1999 10713868	Prospective cohort	Per protocol	CXR	Coexisting disease	None	3569	90 (3%)	<0.01
					Cardiac disease	472	14 (5%)	
					Respiratory disease	207	43 (21%)	
Surgery severity								
Silvestri 1999 10713868	Prospective cohort	Per protocol	CXR	Surgery severity	Major	659	66 (10%)	<0.01
					Minor	870	32 (4%)	
					Standard	4529	215 (5%)	
Surgery type								
Silvestri 1999 10713868	Prospective cohort	Per protocol	CXR	Surgery type	Cardiac	18	2 (11%)	<0.01
					General	1860	112 (6%)	
					Gynecologic	527	14 (3%)	
					Maxillofacial	73	5 (7%)	
					Neurosurgery	121	9 (1%)	
					Ophthalmology	546	16 (3%)	
					Orthopedic	1367	62 (5%)	
					Obstetric	74	1 (1%)	
					Ear, Nose, & Throat	419	3 (1%)	
					Plastic	119	9 (8%)	
					Thoracic	65	21 (32%)	
					Urologic	459	37 (8%)	
					Vascular	225	23 (10%)	

ASA = American Surgical Association; CBC = complete blood count; CXR = chest x ray; ECG = electrocardiogram; NR = not reported
* See Appendix Table C-4 for details of the tests given for each arm.

53

Discussion

Key Findings and Strength of Evidence

We identified 57 studies that reported clinically pertinent outcomes in patients who had routine or per protocol preoperative testing performed. However, only 14 of the studies provided direct comparisons between routine or per protocol testing and ad hoc or no testing, and only two studies compared routine with per protocol testing. Furthermore, only seven of the comparative studies were RCTs, three of which were conducted in patients undergoing cataract surgery. The large majority of data come from cohort studies that provided evidence only about how frequently procedures or anesthesia were canceled, delayed, or altered in response to preoperative testing.

In summary, there is a high strength of evidence from three well-conducted RCTs, that consistently found that for patients scheduled for cataract surgery, preoperative ECG, metabolic panel (or glucose), and CBC have no effect on total perioperative complications or procedure cancellation (Table 17). In contrast, there is insufficient evidence for the effect of routine preoperative testing in all other surgeries and populations. There is also insufficient evidence to estimate a difference in outcomes based on whether preoperative testing was conducted routinely or per protocol. There are one RCT and five nonrandomized studies of routine or per protocol testing in adults undergoing various elective surgeries; however, these studies were highly heterogeneous in populations, elective surgeries, and tests used. Four of these studies compared routine or per protocol testing with ad hoc testing, but in the only one of these studies to report rates of testing, tests were generally ordered *more* frequently in the ad hoc group. Since the true effect of routine (or per protocol) testing can be assessed only when compared with no (or limited) testing, these studies add little to any answer about the effectiveness of routine testing. Furthermore, the nonrandomized studies were all fundamentally flawed in that they failed to adjust for differences among study groups in the patients, surgeries, surgeons, anesthetics used, anesthesiologists, or other possible confounders. These studies generally found lower rates of postoperative complications and deaths among patients undergoing routine or per protocol testing, but the heterogeneity and flaws in the studies preclude any confidence in the accuracy or validity of the findings. However, while there is no evidence regarding minimally invasive surgeries similar to cataract surgery, it may be valid to conclude that routine preoperative testing in these other low-risk surgeries would also have no effect.

There is insufficient evidence for all other categories of procedures and patients, for all other outcomes of interest, and regarding more detailed analyses of differences in how testing is performed. In particular, there is no comparative evidence regarding quality of life or satisfaction, resource utilization, or harms. Among comparative studies, there is insufficient reported evidence regarding how outcomes may differ in different subgroups of patients, or how the effect of preoperative testing may vary based on the risk of the surgical procedure, or other factors.

The apparent difference in the effect of routine or per protocol testing in patients undergoing cataract and general elective surgery is arguably not surprising. Cataract surgery is a very low risk procedure, safe enough to be done in an ophthalmologist's office, that is minimally invasive and usually requires only local anesthesia with sedation. Other than increases in vagal tone, there is little reason to expect cardiac strain in the typical patient undergoing cataract surgery. While the patients are typically elderly, and thus have a relatively high rate of comorbidities, they are generally not suffering from any acute illnesses. In contrast, general elective surgeries in adults encompass a wide range of patients and surgeries, including many with acute or serious medical conditions and highly invasive cardiothoracic, abdominal, and vascular surgeries. These patients are intrinsically at higher risk of perioperative complications and thus, conceptually, may benefit more from preoperative tests that pick up correctable abnormalities that may be associated with complications.

Most of the evidence was from cohort studies. However, the nature of the intervention under consideration (preoperative testing) makes the lack of a direct comparator (no testing) among these studies particularly problematic in terms of interpreting the findings. Regardless of the specific preoperative tests used or how they are implemented, the rate of perioperative complications, due to either the procedure or the anesthesia, will always depend primarily on the underlying risks of the surgical procedure, the type of anesthesia used, the skill and experience of the surgeons and anesthesiologists, the medical condition of the patients, and the quality of perioperative care. The risk of perioperative complications when preoperative testing was conducted, without information about the risk of complications without testing (or only ad hoc testing), does not provide information on the effect of testing on those risks. An adequate comparator is needed that controls for the myriad other factors that impact perioperative complications.

Study Limitations

Across nonrandomized studies, there was a lack of adjustment for possible confounders. They all failed to control for cluster effects, particularly those related to individual surgeons or surgical experience. Six of the nonrandomized studies compared different time periods within an institution before or after implementation or removal of a preoperative testing policy. Furthermore, institutional differences between the time periods (such as incremental improvements in surgical techniques, anesthesia, or nursing care) were not accounted for. The bias that can result from the lack of adjustment (e.g., by propensity score) was best exemplified in the nonrandomized study that compared concurrent surgeries. In one of the two comparative studies comparing routine versus per protocol testing with hemostasis tests on children undergoing tonsillectomy and/or adenoidectomy, the comparison was really between the bleeding complication rates of the 2 most experienced surgeons (who used a testing protocol in 2624 children) and those of the 11 less experienced surgeons (who did routine testing in 1750 children total). Arguably, the finding that perioperative bleeding was more common in the latter group provides evidence that surgical experience and skill are predictors of complications and says little or nothing about whether preoperative testing may (or may not) have prevented any bleeding episodes.

Intrinsic Limitations of Research on Preoperative Testing

Another limitation of the evidence that would be difficult to overcome also relates to the nature of the intervention. Preoperative testing does not in and of itself affect the outcomes of interest (except resource utilization and possibly quality of life/satisfaction, although there are no data on these outcomes). Instead, the preoperative tests potentially cause the health care providers to alter a patient's management—by implementing an intervention to correct or account for the abnormal test; by delaying, canceling, or changing the procedure or anesthesia; or by making changes to postoperative care. Additionally, the preoperative test may be useful for perioperative management to use as a reference (e.g., to know whether a measure has changed in a postoperative test compared with the preoperative test—for example, whether an ECG abnormality is new or not). Thus, the value of any preoperative test is fully dependent on the health care providers and their response to abnormal tests. One could expect responses to vary among surgeons, anesthesiologists, primary care physicians, nurse practitioners, and other providers. One could also expect them to vary among individual providers across hospitals, settings (e.g., urban vs. rural), geographic regions, and a myriad of other health care provider variables. However, none of these factors were accounted for in the studies. This limitation further hampers the interpretation of the evidence, particularly from the cohort studies, but also arguably from the unadjusted nonrandomized studies.

Interpretation of the evidence is further complicated by the wide variability in clinical practice in the thoroughness of preoperative H&P (and whether it is done) and the general lack of reporting regarding H&P in the studies. This could have an important impact on what tests are conducted ad hoc (i.e., in the comparator arms of the studies). Rather than leading to more or less testing, it can lead to more appropriate testing since the tendency to order tests based on a "shotgun" approach will be reduced. But H&P could be considered equivalent to a "test" performed by the clinician (instead of the laboratory or radiology technician), which may—or may not—have value independent of true preoperative tests. Furthermore, H&P is intrinsically nonstandardized and heterogeneous depending on the specific questions asked and the details of the examination. Traditionally, H&Ps have been completed in the surgical clinics and on the day of surgery by the anesthesiology teams. More recently, preoperative assessment clinics staffed by perioperative medicine specialists are becoming more common. These clinics focus on optimizing patients for their perioperative course, and a thorough H&P is the cornerstone of that process. However, none of the studies specifically investigated testing in this setting and none of the studies compared different locations or protocols of care.

Any management changes due to abnormal test results (and presumably any subsequent changes in perioperative outcomes) would be the same regardless of whether testing was done routinely, per protocol, or at the clinician's discretion. Therefore, the variability in ad hoc testing could have an important impact on the comparison of outcomes between ad hoc and routine or per protocol testing. Without good descriptions in studies of typical H&P or the triggers to order ad hoc tests, it is difficult to interpret the applicability of the studies to the general (or any specific) population and the comparison among different testing regimens. Likewise, variations in how abnormal test results are handled at different surgical centers or based on different types of surgery will have a direct impact on the potential effect of preoperative testing. If an abnormal test result is less likely to be acted on in some settings, the value of testing will be reduced in those settings. However, unless centers where studies are conducted use a rigorously followed protocol for posttesting care and other centers follow similar protocols, it may not be possible to overcome this limitation to the applicability of any research into routine preoperative testing.

Limitations of Cohort Studies

Because of the underlying lack of interpretability of the complication rates in these studies, we restricted analyses to "process" outcomes related to decisions about whether the procedure or anesthesia was altered based on testing. These included cancellation or delay of surgery, changes in either the planned surgery or anesthesia, and overall changes in patient management. To the extent possible, based on the reported data, we focused on decisions that were made specifically because of test results (presumably abnormal results), but most studies did not clearly define their outcomes, requiring us to assume this was the case. However, the information to be gleaned from most of these studies was limited. When no procedures were canceled or delayed and no changes were made to either the planned procedure or anesthesia, it may be reasonable to conclude that the testing was of no value at least up to the time that the procedure was performed. However, the assumption that the testing was of no value overall requires that the postoperative course also be unaffected by the availability of the preoperative tests. In reality, it is likely that some abnormal preoperative tests, such as an elevated glucose, would alter perioperative management, such as more intensive glucose monitoring.

Interpreting the finding that a certain (nonzero) percentage of procedures were canceled, delayed, or changed is not straightforward. First, one must make a conclusion as to whether the cancellations, delays, or changes were warranted. Second, one must make assumptions about whether the patients' outcomes were changed. If a procedure was canceled or delayed, at a certain level the patient's immediate health care was worsened, assuming the planned surgery was necessary. However, it is unknowable whether the delay or cancellation may have prevented a complication that would have been worse than the prolongation of the disease state necessitating surgery. Third, one must make a determination as to whether the testing led to changes in care sufficiently rarely (below some percentage threshold) that the testing is of sufficiently limited value to safely forego it, or whether the changes in care occur frequently enough that they can be assumed to be an important tool or predictor regarding surgical management.

With these caveats, the following conclusions can be made from the cohort studies. In all preoperative testing scenarios for which more than a single study was available (i.e., approaching a sufficient evidence base to form a conclusion), testing resulted in some changes in management. In other words, the evidence suggests that in most situations, routine preoperative testing will result in some delay or cancellation of the procedure or some change to anesthetic management or surgical procedure. However, it is not possible to say whether the changes led to benefit or harm for patients. That said, the only studies that directly compared outcomes in subsets of patients were cohort studies that evaluated change in patient management, including specialty consultations or nonsurgery-related changes in patient care. Two studies suggest that change in management from CXR is more common for older patients (primarily >60 years), and one study each suggests that the effect of ECG is similar in men and women, but that CXR results in change in management in more men, those with higher ASA category, those with respiratory disease, and those with "major" surgeries planned (as opposed to "minor" or other surgeries), particularly in patients undergoing thoracic, cardiac, and vascular surgeries. Two studies suggest that change in management from CXR is more common for older patients (primarily >60 years). Two studies also looked at CXR and ECG by sex and other factors. One of these studies suggests that the effect of ECG is similar in men and women, but the second study suggests that CXR results in change in management in more men, those in a higher ASA risk category, those with respiratory disease, and those with "major" surgeries planned (as opposed to "minor" or "standard" surgeries), particularly in patients undergoing thoracic, cardiac, and vascular surgeries. However, given the small number of studies that compared outcomes in different subgroups of patients, together with the unknown connection between changing patient management and true patient outcomes, it is premature to conclude that the differences found are clinically important.

There is no comparative evidence regarding quality of life or satisfaction, changes in anesthesia or procedure, resource utilization, or harms. Among comparative studies, there is no (or insufficient) reported evidence regarding how outcomes may differ in different subgroups of patients (e.g., based on age, sex, medical status, or anesthesia risk category) or how the effect of preoperative testing may vary based on the risk of the surgical procedure, the type of anesthesia planned, the indication for surgery, who orders or responds to the results of the preoperative tests, whether testing is done routinely (in everyone) or per protocol, or the length of time prior to the planned procedures that the tests are conducted.

Table 17. Routine or per protocol preoperative testing: Findings and strength of evidence

Outcome	Surgery	Tests	Study Design (Risk of Bias)	Finding	Strength of Evidence
Perioperative complications, total	Cataract surgery	ECG, metabolic panel, CBC	RCT (2 low, 1 medium)	No effect of testing. Summary RR=0.99; 95% CI 0.86, 1.14)	High
	Various, adults (comparison: routine vs. ad hoc testing)	Multiple*	RCT (1 low) NRS (4 high)	In most studies, fewer complications occurred with testing, but studies were highly heterogeneous and underpowered; not a clinically important difference	Insufficient
	Various, adults (comparison: routine vs. per protocol testing	Multiple*	NRS (1 high)	No events in either group.	Insufficient
	Various, children	Multiple†	NRS (1 high)	More complications occurred with testing, but not a clinically important difference	Insufficient
	Vascular, adults	Stress echo	RCT (1 high)	No significant difference in cardiac events	Insufficient
Perioperative death	Various, adults (comparison: routine vs. ad hoc testing)	Multiple*	NRS (4 high)	In most studies, fewer deaths occurred with testing, but studies were highly heterogeneous and underpowered	Insufficient
	Various, adults (comparison: routine vs. per protocol testing	Multiple*	NRS (1 high)	No events in either group.	Insufficient
	Vascular, adults	Stress echo	RCT (1 high)	Cardiac and respiratory deaths were rare, no difference between groups	Insufficient
Perioperative complications, major (total)	Various, children	Multiple†	NRS (1 high)	Imprecise estimate failing to support a difference.	Insufficient

Table 17. Routine or per protocol preoperative testing: Findings and strength of evidence (continued)

Outcome	Surgery	Tests	Study Design (Risk of Bias)	Finding	Strength of Evidence
Perioperative complications, specific (selected)	Various, adults (comparison: routine vs. ad hoc testing)	Multiple*	RCT (1 low) NRS (3 high)	Clinically important difference: fewer episodes of renal failure with testing (0.9% vs. 0%; 1 study). Significant but not clinically important difference: fewer episodes of pneumonia with testing (1 study). No significant differences for other complications, including any outcome from RCT.	Insufficient
	Various, adults (comparison: routine vs. per protocol testing	Multiple*	NRS (1 high)	No difference between groups, but only rare events.	Insufficient
	Various, children	Multiple†	NRS (1 high)	Clinically important more episodes of persistent vomiting with testing (RR=1.76; 95% CI 1.22, 2.54). Clinically important more episodes of restlessness with testing (RR=3.91; 95% CI 2.19, 6.97). No significant differences were found for other complications.	Insufficient
	Tonsillectomy, children (comparison: routine vs. ad hoc testing)	Coagulation tests	NRS (1 high)	No significant difference in bleeding complications	Insufficient
Return to operating room	Various, adults	Multiple*	NRS (1 high)	No significant difference in rate of return to operating room	Insufficient
Unplanned hospital admission	Orthopedic, adults	Multiple*	NRS (1 high)	No significant difference in rate of unplanned hospital admissions	Insufficient

60

Table 17. Routine or per protocol preoperative testing: Findings and strength of evidence (continued)

Outcome	Surgery	Tests	Study Design (Risk of Bias)	Finding	Strength of Evidence
Procedure cancellation	Cataract surgery	ECG, metabolic panel, CBC	RCT (1 low, 1 medium)	Likely no effect of testing‡ Summary RR=0.97 (95% CI 0.79, 1.20)	High
	Various, adults	Multiple*	NRS (1 high)	Possibly no effect of testing. RR= 0.93 (95% CI 0.76, 1.14)	Insufficient
	Various, children	Multiple†	NRS (1 high)	No effect of testing (no surgeries canceled).	Insufficient
Procedure delay	Various, adults	Multiple*	NRS (1 high)	No significant difference in procedure delay	Insufficient
Length of stay	Various, adults	Multiple*	NRS (1 high)	No significant difference in length of stay	Insufficient
	Various, children	Multiple†	RCT (1 medium) NRS (1 high)	No significant difference in length of stay	Insufficient
Quality of life/Satisfaction Anesthesia change Surgery change Resource utilization Harms	None	Not applicable	No studies	None	Insufficient
Subgroup analyses	None	Not applicable	No studies	None	Insufficient

CBC = complete blood count; CI = confidence interval; ECG = electrocardiogram; NRS = nonrandomized comparative study; RCT=randomized controlled trial; RR = relative risk; stress echo = dobutamine stress echocardiogram.

* ECG, CXR, basic and extended metabolic panels, CBC, coagulation tests, and urinalysis

† Hemoglobin, urinalysis, creatinine phosphokinase, and cholinesterase

‡ Just fails to meet 20% MID threshold for evidence of no difference.

61

Limitations of Systematic Review

We relied mainly on electronic database searches and perusal of reference lists to identify relevant studies. Unpublished relevant studies may have been missed. We also kept the review focused on the evidence that most directly addresses the comparative effect of routine (or per protocol) preoperative testing versus ad hoc or no testing. Thus, we did not review the wide range of indirect evidence from which conclusions about whether testing might be of value might be inferred. The Statement of Work in the Introduction spells out the broader research questions that were not addressed here. The decision to narrow the scope of the review was made in part due to time and resource constraints. Future updates of this review may be able to broaden the scope of the research questions, particularly if it remains the case that there are few eligible comparative studies.

The conclusions, to a large extent, reflect the limitations of the underlying evidence base. Our ability to address most of the issues raised by the Key Questions was hampered by a paucity, or complete lack, of data, particularly from comparative studies.

Applicability

The applicability of the evidence is limited, with the exception of the studies of cataract surgery. The cataract RCTs had similar findings, despite being conducted in different settings, in different countries, and with somewhat different eligibility criteria and study designs. Furthermore, the first trial was conducted in nearly 20,000 patients. This all implies that the conclusion that there is no effect of routine testing with ECG, a basic metabolic panel, and blood counts for cataract surgery is likely to be broadly applicable. The applicability of the findings for adults undergoing a range of elective surgeries is less clear. The studies evaluated different tests in different populations receiving different surgical procedures and did not adequately report the conditions under which ad hoc testing was done (i.e., the extent of H&P or the triggers to order testing).

Comparison With Prior Systematic Reviews and Guidelines

In 2003, the United Kingdom-based NICE published the only prior broad evidence review (with a guideline) we identified that addresses these Key Questions.[9] We included all studies identified in the NICE review that met our eligibility criteria. In contrast with our review, which was structured to identify which patients undergoing which procedures could benefit (or be harmed) by routine testing, the NICE review was structured by test, regardless of procedure or patient characteristics. The principal difference in conclusions between NICE and the current review relates to tests for cataract surgery, since two of the three trials we used were not published until after the NICE review was conducted. Otherwise, the NICE review was similar in that it found insufficient evidence. Specifically, it found that the evidence could not directly inform their guideline for CXR, ECG, CBC, hemostasis tests, biochemistry tests, urinalysis, pregnancy tests, sickle cell testing, or pulmonary function testing. A Health Technology Assessment subsequent to the NICE review conducted a limited systematic review in 2008 (published in 2012) of blood and pulmonary function tests in low- or medium-risk patients,[10] but included no studies comparing testing versus no testing. A recent Cochrane review focused on

RCTs of routine preoperative testing for cataract surgery and came to the same conclusion found here, based on the same studies we included.[11]

The American College of Physicians wrote an evidence-based guideline in 2006 on preoperative testing to reduce perioperative pulmonary complications for patients undergoing noncardiothoracic surgery.[83] The associated systematic review evaluated patient- and procedure-related risk factors and laboratory predictors of postoperative pulmonary complication rates.[84] Their conclusions are based primarily on 27 studies with multivariable analyses, but they also included 83 studies with univariable data. However, they did not consider whether testing was done routinely, per protocol, or ad hoc. Given the state of the evidence, the guideline recommendations for which tests to use or not use in which patients are based on whether various predictors have been associated with pulmonary complications, as opposed to whether routine or per protocol testing has been found to reduce or mitigate pulmonary complications.

The ACC/AHA also wrote an evidence-based guideline (in 2007) on perioperative cardiovascular evaluation prior to noncardiac surgery.[12] The committee reviewed more than 400 new articles (since 2002) on a broad range of topics, including preoperative evaluation, perioperative and cardiac risk and complications, and noncardiac surgery. Among several topics they covered on perioperative management, they provide recommendations on stepwise noninvasive and invasive cardiac testing based on patients' risk factors and symptoms, Although, the guideline does not specify the evidence used for each recommendation, all recommendations are level B or C meaning that the recommendations are based on either single comparative studies, a small number of conflicting comparative studies, or on expert opinion. Apparently, the guideline did not rely on comparative studies of the effect of routine or per protocol testing since only one of the comparative studies (on cataract surgery[85]) eligible for this review was cited in the guideline.

In 2012, the ASA reported an updated practice advisory for preanesthesia evaluation.[1] They issued a practice advisory, as opposed to a guideline, "because of the lack of sufficient numbers of adequately controlled trials."[1] They systematically searched for studies with "evidence linkages, consisting of directional statements about relationships among specific preanesthesia evaluation activities and clinical outcomes" that could assess causality. They found no studies that met their criteria, so they also reviewed "descriptive literature" (reports of frequency or incidence) and case reports. All of their advisories about the use of specific tests were based on noncomparative observational studies with associative or descriptive statistics, i.e., not on evidence regarding the comparative effect of routine or per protocol testing.

Ongoing Research

A search on July 11, 2013 in the ClinicalTrials.gov registry (of "preoperative," "presurgical," "preprocedural," and related terms) identified only one potentially relevant record of a study that would meet eligibility criteria for this review. The study, whose status is "unknown," plans to compare the use of cardiac stress tests or no testing in patients undergoing colorectal surgery. They plan to report on patient outcomes, patient satisfaction, and resource usage.[a]

---

[a] Cardiopulmonary Exercise Testing and Preoperative Risk Stratification (CPX or CPEX). ClinicalTrials.gov Identifier: NCT00737828.

Evidence Gaps

Table 18 summarizes the evidence gaps with regard to the two Key Questions and subquestions of this systematic review.

Table 18. Evidence gaps

Key Question	Category	Evidence Gap
Beneficial effects of routine or per protocol preoperative testing	General	For all procedures and surgeries requiring more than local anesthesia, except cataract surgery, there is a paucity or lack of comparative studies to assess the value of the intervention.
	Population	Evidence is needed to evaluate the effect of testing for All elective procedures except cataract surgery Specific procedures Different types of anesthesia Different aged populations—children, adults, and older adults Different preoperative health status, including comorbidities Different categories of anesthesia risk Existing studies generally provide poor descriptions of the patient populations—specific procedures planned, disease conditions, comorbidities, surgical and anesthesia risk categories, race, and other factors.
	Interventions and comparators	Difference in effect of routine testing (in all patients) vs. per protocol testing (in selected patients). Effect of individual tests (within panels of tests) compared with effect of other individual tests. Different effects based on who ordered the test or the structure of testing (e.g., if done through a preanesthesia clinic or internist's office). These data are generally not reported. How long prior to the planned procedure tests can be performed (e.g., within 1 week or 6-12 months) and still provide a benefit (assuming the preoperative testing is beneficial).
	Outcomes	Major perioperative complications (to some degree in contrast with total complications). Quality of life or satisfaction. Resource utilization. Postoperative management. Perioperative complications: improved standardization is needed regarding which perioperative complications should be reported; however, the list of complications will vary depending on the procedure.
Harms of routine or per protocol preoperative testing	General / outcomes	There is no evidence regarding harms of testing.
Subgroup analyses	General	No comparative studies provided subgroup analyses based on any baseline patient characteristics, procedures, anesthesia type, or other factors listed above under Population or Interventions and comparators.

Future Research

As noted above, this review identified major gaps in the published evidence on the comparative effectiveness and safety of routine and per protocol preoperative testing. We believe that the following evidence gaps can be fruitful areas for future research:

- *RCTs to evaluate the comparative effectiveness of preoperative testing:* RCTs remains the best study design to minimize bias. A common complaint about RCTs is that they have limited applicability, largely due to their narrow scope. However, the current nonrandomized studies have limited applicability because they are too inclusive and do not adequately account for vast heterogeneity of elective procedures, potential tests, information about typical H&P, triggers for ad hoc testing, processes for obtaining and handling the test results, and patients themselves. More focused studies evaluating specific tests or panels of tests in well-defined patients undergoing a narrow set of procedures will be of greater value to clinicians and decisionmakers deciding who should be routinely tested preoperatively. RCTs are of particular value in evaluating preoperative testing to maximize the likelihood of balancing patients between groups. In all studies, regardless of design, confounding will be a particularly important analytic concern, especially as it relates to the likelihood of both abnormal test results and perioperative complications based on a patient's age, comorbidities, and other characteristics. Again, RCTs can best minimize allocation bias and confounding. If the current RCT evidence from cataract surgery is considered to be sufficiently convincing by ophthalmologists, hospitals, payers, and other policymakers, then an argument can be made that no further RCTs are needed to investigate the value of routine preoperative ECGs, basic metabolic panel, or complete blood count. However, given that there is only a single 38 year old RCT for any other procedure (pediatric elective surgery), RCTs for all other procedures, in all populations, and for all specific tests are warranted. Conducting a series of such trials appears to be quite feasible, given the large number of elective procedures performed at many hospitals (or surgical clinics), the low cost of the intervention (since in many situations the trial will primarily involve randomizing patients to either receive tests that are already available to them or withholding those tests, as opposed to requiring resources to cover the costs of additional interventions), and that only a short-term postoperative followup is required (during hospitalization or up to 1 to 3 months). Somewhat more complex trials to organize upfront, cluster randomized trials, where centers or units are randomized as opposed to individual patients, can also provide informative data, provided that they are analyzed appropriately. Cluster randomized trials may be easier to run since the randomization procedure is much simpler. Trials should collect sufficient data to effectively stratify patients based on the major variables of interest (procedures, tests, comorbidities, etc.) or alternatively, multiple trials should be run, each focused on a specific aspect of the research question. In particular, since it is likely that the effect of preoperative testing will vary substantially based on the specific surgery (as suggested by the different effects found between cataract trials and general surgery studies), trials should either focus on a single type of surgery or, at a minimum, stratify their results by surgery or surgery risk class. Furthermore, studies should stratify their results based on patient risk category, such as ASA category, and comorbidities. They should capture the full range of perioperative outcomes, including patient quality of life/satisfaction and resource utilization. They should be sufficiently powered to evaluate, at a minimum, total major perioperative complications. Preferably they should be sufficiently powered to cover specific major complications, such as death. They should also be sufficiently powered to allow for a priori subgroup analyses and analyses specific to (at least some) individual procedures and tests.

- o Likely, the major hurdle in conducting new RCTs is that there is no private source of funding (e.g., pharmaceutical or device manufacturers) since, by definition, preoperative tests are common, universally available tests. However, we believe that finding the balance between maximizing periprocedural risk and harm reduction and minimizing wasteful resource utilization ought to make this question of interest to funders and policymakers.

- *Observational studies for the comparative effectiveness of preoperative testing:* Observational studies can provide a lesser level of evidence to provide information on the comparative effectiveness of alternative preoperative testing strategies. However, the intrinsic heterogeneity and risk of confounding requires that great care and attention be given to how the data are analyzed (e.g., with a priori subgroup analyses) and whether it is possible to adequately adjust for fundamental differences among nonrandomized cohorts of patients having or not having testing done. At a minimum, observational studies need to be adjusted for differences in patient and surgical characteristics and to control for cluster effects of individual surgeons or based on surgical experience. The common approach used by nonrandomized comparative studies to date is to compare patients before and after a hospital policy change. However, these analyses are subject to temporal trend biases, where patient care changes over time in multiple ways independent of the change in testing policy, and these changes are unknown, cannot be quantified, or cannot be otherwise adequately adjusted for. A few examples include the use of new surgical equipment, changes in surgical techniques and training, and changes in the health status of the patients. To be of use, observational studies should include concurrent patients who do or do not receive testing and who are as similar as possible. Even then, it will be important to use strong statistical methods to adjust analyses for differences in the cohorts unrelated to testing and confounders (e.g., propensity score or instrumental variable methods). Quantitative bias analyses could be used to address concerns regarding unobserved confounding in nonrandomized studies. Although the use of observational data always requires additional assumptions for valid inference on treatment effects (compared to randomized designs), well designed observational studies may be able to offer valuable information regarding the effectiveness and adverse effects of routine or per protocol preoperative testing. All the suggestions made for RCTs regarding focusing or stratifying analyses based on surgical, patient, and other study characteristics also apply to observational studies.

- *Decision models:* In the face of a paucity of reliable evidence regarding the benefits, harms, and resources used with routine or per protocol preoperative testing, decision analyses may be of value to delineate plausible estimates of the range of how beneficial (or harmful) and resource-intensive preoperative testing could be. Such analyses could be useful to rank tests and procedures by likely benefit and thus help to prioritize research for specific tests and procedures. Such models will require direct evidence of the comparative effect of testing, as reviewed here, along with other indirect evidence including the likelihood of (specific) perioperative complications (for specific procedures), the likelihood that specific tests will diagnose conditions that would impact the rate of complications, the effects of correcting or ameliorating any such conditions, whether a test result could be acted on to impact the rate of complications, the likelihood of true and false positive test results, and the effects of delaying or canceling the procedures.

Regardless of the design of future studies, to allow answers to the main question of the value of routine (or per protocol) preoperative testing, it is important that a large number of studies be conducted covering a wide range of scenarios, but that they are specific enough to allow applicability for decisions to be made for particular patients undergoing particular procedures in a given setting. These various scenarios include differences in patient populations (e.g., by age, comorbidities, and other risk factors), procedures (e.g., either specific surgeries or categories of procedures by risk), tests that may be of benefit (depending on patient and procedure), differences in how testing typically occurs and the triggers for ad hoc testing, who orders and follows up on test results, surgical center type and setting, timing of the testing, and so forth. Alternative prioritization approaches may be reasonable. Initially focusing on people who are most likely to have life-threatening perioperative complications, including older patients, those in higher ASA categories, those with important comorbidities, and those undergoing higher-risk surgeries would allow for relatively small, low-resource, studies that would be adequately powered. In these cases, complications would be more common and test abnormalities may also be more common. Not only would studies of these groups have the greatest potential to affect patients most likely to have complications, but the studies would also be better powered due to the higher complication rates than in lower-risk populations. Further studies of patients at high risk of surgical bleeding (for example children undergoing tonsillectomy and/or adenoidectomy) are also warranted. Alternatively, one could argue that future research should focus on lower-risk populations and surgeries (e.g., Grades 1, 2, and possibly 3 surgeries; see Table 1). While these studies would need to be relatively large, due to low complication rates, the findings of these studies may have the greatest impact since they would address more common surgeries and more typical patients. Furthermore, hospitals, clinicians, and patients may be more willing to forgo preoperative testing in low- rather than high-risk settings. We believe it is likely that higher-risk patients undergoing higher-risk procedures would continue to have preoperative testing done regardless of evidence showing the testing to be ineffective. Given the different arguments that could be made about who to include in future studies, and limited resources to conduct such research, this topic may be worthy of undergoing a formal value of information analysis.[86]

Given the large number of elective procedures performed annually in the U.S. and the large number of tests that can be ordered routinely, further data are needed regarding resource utilization. Both RCTs (either within centers or cluster randomized across centers) and observational studies can provide useful information on costs of tests, costs of changes in management (including delay or cancellation), costs of followup testing and treatment, and costs of complications.

Conclusions

With the exception of cataract surgery, there is a paucity of reliable evidence regarding the benefits, harms, and resource utilization associated with routine or per protocol preoperative testing for all tests used for all procedures. There is a high strength of evidence, which is broadly applicable, that ECG, basic metabolic panel (biochemistry), and CBC have no effect on important clinical outcomes in patients scheduled for cataract surgery, including total perioperative complications and procedure cancellations. But despite several nonrandomized studies, there is insufficient evidence regarding the value of routine or per protocol preoperative testing for other procedures and populations. Based on studies with a high risk of bias, there is a possibility that complications and deaths occurred more commonly among patients undergoing ad hoc as opposed to routine or per protocol testing. This raises a caution against extrapolating the cataract findings to other surgeries and populations who may be at higher risk of complications due to the nature of the procedures or underlying illnesses and comorbidities. The evidence is insufficient to clarify specifically which routinely conducted (or per protocol) tests may be of benefit (or no benefit) for which patients undergoing which procedures. There is insufficient evidence to make conclusions related to the effect of routine versus per protocol testing. There is no evidence regarding quality of life or satisfaction, resource utilization, or harms of testing. There is also no evidence regarding how the value of testing may differ based on the risks of a specific surgical procedure, the type of anesthesia planned, the indication for surgery, comorbidities or other patient characteristics, the structure of testing (e.g., whether ordered through a specialized preoperative clinic), by who orders the tests (e.g., surgeon vs. anesthesiologist vs. primary care physician), or the length of time prior to the procedure that the tests are conducted. Given the large number of patients undergoing elective surgery, there is a clear need to develop better evidence for when routine or per protocol testing improves patient outcomes and what the harms may be.

References

1. Apfelbaum JL, Connis RT, Nickinovich DG, et al. Practice advisory for preanesthesia evaluation: an updated report by the American Society of Anesthesiologists Task Force on Preanesthesia Evaluation. Anesthesiology. 2012 Mar;116(3):522-38. PMID: 22273990.

2. Kumar A, Srivastava U. Role of routine laboratory investigations in preoperative evaluation. J Anaesthesiol Clin Pharmacol. 2011 Apr;27(2):174-79. PMID: 21772675.

3. Bryson GL. Has preoperative testing become a habit? Can J Anaesth. 2005 Jun;52(6):557-61. PMID: 15983138.

4. Kaplan EB, Sheiner LB, Boeckmann AJ, et al. The usefulness of preoperative laboratory screening. JAMA. 1985 Jun 28;253(24):3576-81. PMID: 3999339.

5. Johnson RK, Mortimer AJ. Routine pre-operative blood testing: is it necessary? Anaesthesia. 2002 Sep;57(9):914-17. PMID: 12190758.

6. Pasternak LR. Preoperative testing: moving from individual testing to risk management. Anesth Analg. 2009 Feb;108(2):393-94. PMID: 19151262.

7. MacPherson RD, Reeve SA, Stewart TV, et al. Effective strategy to guide pathology test ordering in surgical patients. ANZ J Surg. 2005 Mar;75(3):138-43. PMID: 15777393.

8. Klein AA, Arrowsmith JE. Should routine pre-operative testing be abandoned? Anaesthesia. 2010 Oct;65(10):974-76. PMID: 21198466.

9. National Collaborating Centre for Acute Care (UK). Preoperative Tests: The use of routine preoperative tests for elective surgery. London: National Institute for Health and Clinical Excellence: Guidance; 2003. PMID: 21089235.

10. Czoski-Murray C, Lloyd Jones M, McCabe C, et al. What is the value of routinely testing full blood count, electrolytes and urea, and pulmonary function tests before elective surgery in patients with no apparent clinical indication and in subgroups of patients with common comorbidities: a systematic review of the clinical and cost-effective literature. Health Techol Assess. 2012;16(50):1-159. PMID: 23302507.

11. Keay L, Lindsley K, Tielsch J, et al. Routine preoperative medical testing for cataract surgery. Cochrane Database of Systematic Reviews. 2012(3):CD0079293.

12. Fleisher LA, Beckman JA, Brown KA, et al. ACC/AHA 2007 Guidelines on Perioperative Cardiovascular Evaluation and Care for Noncardiac Surgery: Executive Summary: A Report of the American College of Cardiology/American Heart Association Task Force on Practice Guidelines (Writing Committee to Revise the 2002 Guidelines on Perioperative Cardiovascular Evaluation for Noncardiac Surgery) Developed in Collaboration With the American Society of Echocardiography, American Society of Nuclear Cardiology, Heart Rhythm Society, Society of Cardiovascular Anesthesiologists, Society for Cardiovascular Angiography and Interventions, Society for Vascular Medicine and Biology, and Society for Vascular Surgery. J Am Coll Cardiol. 2007 Oct 23;50(17):1707-32. PMID: 17950159.

13. American College of Radiology. ACR Appropriateness Criteria: Routine Admission and Preoperative Chest Radiography. http://www.acr.org/~/media/ACR/Documents/AppCriteria/Diagnostic/RoutineAdmissionAndPreoperativeChestRadiography.pdf. 2013

14. American Society of Anesthesiologists. ASA Physical Status Classification System. http://www.asahq.org/Home/For-Members/Clinical-Information/ASA-Physical-Status-Classification-System. Last accessed 7/1/2013.

15. Wallace BW, Small K, Brodley CE, et al. Deploying an interactive machine learning system in an evidence-based practice center: Abstrackr. Proceedings of the ACM International Health Informatics Symposium (IHI). 2012:819-24.

16. Owens DK, Lohr KN, Atkins D, et al. AHRQ series paper 5: grading the strength of a body of evidence when comparing medical interventions--agency for healthcare research and quality and the effective health-care program. J Clin Epidemiol. 2010 May;63(5):513-23. PMID: 19595577.

17. Higgins J.P. Cochrane handbook for systematic reviews of interventions. Version 5.0.2. [updated September 2009]. The Cochrane Collaboration. 2009

18. Chou R, Aronson N, Atkins D, et al. AHRQ series paper 4: assessing harms when comparing medical interventions: AHRQ and the effective health-care program. J Clin Epidemiol. 2010 May;63(5):502-12. PMID: 18823754.

19. Santaguida P, Raina P, Ismaila A. McMaster Quality Assessment Scale of Harms (McHarm) for primary studies, http://bmg.cochrane.org/sites/bmg.cochrane.org/files/uploads/McHarm%20for%20Primary%20Studies.pdf, last accessed 1/8/13.

20. DerSimonian R, Laird N. Meta-analysis in clinical trials. Control Clin Trials. 1986 Sep;7(3):177-88. PMID: 3802833.

21. Higgins JP, Thompson SG. Quantifying heterogeneity in a meta-analysis. Stat Med. 2002 Jun 15;21(11):1539-58. PMID: 12111919.

22. Higgins JP, Thompson SG, Deeks JJ, et al. Measuring inconsistency in meta-analyses. BMJ. 2003 Sep 6;327(7414):557-60. PMID: 12958120.

23. Whitlock EP, Lopez SA, Chang S, et al. AHRQ series paper 3: identifying, selecting, and refining topics for comparative effectiveness systematic reviews: AHRQ and the effective health-care program. J Clin Epidemiol. 2010 May;63(5):491-501.

24. Berkman ND, Lohr KN, Ansari Meal. Grading the Strength of a Body of Evidence When Assessing Health Care Interventions for the Effective Health Care Program of the Agency for Healthcare Research and Quality: An Update. Methods Research Report. PENDING. 2013

25. Almanaseer Y, Mukherjee D, Kline-Rogers EM, et al. Implementation of the ACC/AHA guidelines for preoperative cardiac risk assessment in a general medicine preoperative clinic: improving efficiency and preserving outcomes. Cardiology. 2005;103(1):24-29. PMID: 15528897.

26. Cavallini GM, Saccarola P, D'Amico R, et al. Impact of preoperative testing on ophthalmologic and systemic outcomes in cataract surgery. Eur J Ophthalmol. 2004 Sep;14(5):369-74. PMID: 15506597.

27. Finegan BA, Rashiq S, McAlister FA, et al. Selective ordering of preoperative investigations by anesthesiologists reduces the number and cost of tests. Can J Anaesth. 2005 Jun;52(6):575-80. PMID: 15983141.

28. Larocque BJ, Maykut RJ. Implementation of guidelines for preoperative laboratory investigations in patients scheduled to undergo elective surgery. Can J Surg. 1994 Oct;37(5):397-401. PMID: 7922901.

29. Leonard JV, Clayton BE, Colley JR. Use of biochemical profile in children's hospital: results of two controlled trials. Br Med J. 1975 Jun 21;2(5972):662-65. PMID: 1095116.

30. Lira RP, Nascimento MA, Moreira-Filho DC, et al. Are routine preoperative medical tests needed with cataract surgery? Rev Panam Salud Publica. 2001 Jul;10(1):13-17. PMID: 11558245.

31. Nascimento MA, Lira RP, Soares PH, et al. Are routine preoperative medical tests needed with cataract surgery? Study of visual acuity outcome. Curr Eye Res. 2004 Apr;28(4):285-90. PMID: 15259298.

32. Meneghini L, Zadra N, Zanette G, et al. The usefulness of routine preoperative laboratory tests for one-day surgery in healthy children. Paediatr Anaesth. 1998;8(1):11-15. PMID: 9483592.

33. Schein OD, Katz J, Bass EB, et al. The value of routine preoperative medical testing before cataract surgery. Study of Medical Testing for Cataract Surgery. N Engl J Med. 2000 Jan 20;342(3):168-75. PMID: 10639542.

34. Wyatt WJ, Reed DN, Jr., Apelgren KN. Pitfalls in the role of standardized preadmission laboratory screening for ambulatory surgery. Am Surg. 1989 Jun;55(6):343-46.

35. Zwack GC, Derkay CS. The utility of preoperative hemostatic assessment in adenotonsillectomy. Int J Pediatr Otorhinolaryngol. 1997 Feb 14;39(1):67-76. PMID: 9051441.

36. Chung F, Yuan H, Yin L, et al. Elimination of preoperative testing in ambulatory surgery. Anesth Analg. 2009;108(2):467-75. PMID: 19151274.

37. Falcone RA, Nass C, Jermyn R, et al. The value of preoperative pharmacologic stress testing before vascular surgery using ACC/AHA guidelines: a prospective, randomized trial. J Cardiothorac Vasc Anesth. 2003;17(6):694-98. PMID: 14689407.

38. Mancuso CA. Impact of new guidelines on physicians' ordering of preoperative tests. J Gen Intern Med. 1999;14(3):166-72. PMID: 10203622.

39. Mignonsin D, Degui S, Kane M, et al. [Value of selective prescription of preanesthetic laboratory tests]. [French]. Cah Anesthesiol. 1996;44(1):13-17. PMID: 8762245.

40. Aghajanian A, Grimes DA. Routine prothrombin time determination before elective gynecologic operations. Obstet Gynecol. 1991 Nov;78(5:Pt 1):837-39. PMID: 1923209.

41. Alsumait BM, Alhumood SA, Ivanova T, et al. A prospective evaluation of preoperative screening laboratory tests in general surgery patients. Med Princ Pract. 2002 Jan;11(1):42-45. PMID: 12116695.

42. Azzam FJ, Padda GS, DeBoard JW, et al. Preoperative pregnancy testing in adolescents. Anesth Analg. 1996 Jan;82(1):4-7. PMID: 8712424.

43. Baron MJ, Gunter J, White P. Is the pediatric preoperative hematocrit determination necessary? South Med J. 1992 Dec;85(12):1187-89. PMID: 1470961.

44. Bhuripanyo K, Prasertchuang C, Chamadol N, et al. The impact of routine preoperative chest X-ray in Srinagarind Hospital, Khon Kaen. J Med Assoc Thai. 1990 Jan;73(1):21-28. PMID: 2345323.

45. Bhuripanyo K, Prasertchuang C, Viwathanatepa M, et al. The impact of routine preoperative electrocardiogram in patients age > or = 40 years in Srinagarind Hospital. J Med Assoc Thai. 1992 Jul;75(7):399-406. PMID: 1293256.

46. Bhuripanyo K, Khumsuk K, Sornpanya N, et al. The impact of routine preoperative complete blood count (CBC) in elective operations in Srinagarind Hospital. J Med Assoc Thai. 1995 Jan;78(1):42-47. PMID: 7622976.

47. Bhuripanyo K, Prasertchuang C, Khumsuk K, et al. The impact of routine preoperative urinalysis in Srinagarind Hospital, Khon Kaen. J Med Assoc Thai. 1995 Feb;78(2):94-98. PMID: 7629451.

48. Bouillot JL, Fingerhut A, Paquet JC, et al. Are routine preoperative chest radiographs useful in general surgery? A prospective, multicentre study in 3959 patients. Association des Chirurgiens de l'Assistance Publique pour les Evaluations medicales. Eur J Surg. 1996 Aug;162(8):597-604. PMID: 8891616.

49. Burk CD, Miller L, Handler SD, et al. Preoperative history and coagulation screening in children undergoing tonsillectomy. Pediatrics. 1992 Apr;89(4:Pt 2):691-95.

50. Bushick JB, Eisenberg JM, Kinman J, et al. Pursuit of abnormal coagulation screening tests generates modest hidden preoperative costs. J Gen Intern Med. 1989 Nov;4(6):493-97. PMID: 2585157.

51. Carliner NH, Fisher ML, Plotnick GD, et al. The preoperative electrocardiogram as an indicator of risk in major noncardiac surgery. Can J Cardiol. 1986 May;2(3):134-37. PMID: 3719447.

52. Charpak Y, Blery C, Chastang C, et al. Usefulness of selectively ordered preoperative tests. Med Care. 1988 Feb;26(2):95-104. PMID: 3339918.

53. Charpak Y, Blery C, Chastang C, et al. Prospective assessment of a protocol for selective ordering of preoperative chest x-rays. Can J Anaesth. 1988 May;35(3:(Pt 1)):259-64.

54. Correll DJ, Hepner DL, Chang C, et al. Preoperative electrocardiograms: patient factors predictive of abnormalities. Anesthesiology. 2009 Jun;110(6):1217-22. PMID: 19417620.

55. Gabriel P, Mazoit X, Ecoffey C. Relationship between clinical history, coagulation tests, and perioperative bleeding during tonsillectomies in pediatrics. J Clin Anesth. 2000 Jun;12(4):288-91. PMID: 10960200.

56. Gold BS, Young ML, Kinman JL, et al. The utility of preoperative electrocardiograms in the ambulatory surgical patient. Arch Intern Med. 1992 Feb;152(2):301-05. PMID: 1739358.

57. Golub R, Cantu R, Sorrento JJ, et al. Efficacy of preadmission testing in ambulatory surgical patients. Am J Surg. 1992;163(6):565-70. PMID: 1595835.

58. Haug RH, Reifeis RL. A prospective evaluation of the value of preoperative laboratory testing for office anesthesia and sedation. J Oral Maxillofac Surg. 1999 Feb 21;57(1):16-20. PMID: 9915390.

59. Hoare TJ. Pre-operative haemoglobin estimation in paediatric ENT surgery. J Laryngol Otol. 1993 Dec;107(12):1146-48. PMID: 8289005.

60. Ipp L, Flynn P, Blanco J, et al. The findings of preoperative cardiac screening studies in adolescent idiopathic scoliosis. J Pediatr Orthop. 2011 Oct;31(7):764-66. PMID: 21926874.

61. Johnson H, Jr., Knee-Ioli S, Butler TA, et al. Are routine preoperative laboratory screening tests necessary to evaluate ambulatory surgical patients? Surgery. 1988 Oct;104(4):639-45. PMID: 3175862.

62. Kahn RL, Stanton MA, Tong-Ngork S, et al. One-year experience with day-of-surgery pregnancy testing before elective orthopedic procedures. Anesth Analg. 2008;106(4):1127-31. PMID: 18349183.

63. Lafferty JE, North CS, Spitznagel E, et al. Laboratory screening prior to ECT. J ECT. 2001 Sep;17(3):158-65. PMID: 11528304.

64. Lawrence VA, Kroenke K. The unproven utility of preoperative urinalysis. Clinical use. Arch Intern Med. 1988 Jun;148(6):1370-73. PMID: 3377621.

65. Mallick MS. Is routine pre-operative blood testing in children necessary? Saudi Med J. 2006 Dec;27(12):1831-34. PMID: 17143358.

66. Malviya S, D'Errico C, Reynolds P, et al. Should pregnancy testing be routine in adolescent patients prior to surgery? Anesth Analg. 1996 Oct;83(4):854-58. PMID: 8831334.

67. Manning SC, Beste D, McBride T, et al. An assessment of preoperative coagulation screening for tonsillectomy and adenoidectomy. Int J Pediatr Otorhinolaryngol. 1987 Oct;13(3):237-44. PMID: 3679679.

68. Mantha S, Roizen MF, Madduri J, et al. Usefulness of routine preoperative testing: a prospective single-observer study. J Clin Anesth. 2005 Feb;17(1):51-57. PMID: 15721730.

69. Narr BJ, Hansen TR, Warner MA. Preoperative laboratory screening in healthy Mayo patients: cost-effective elimination of tests and unchanged outcomes. Mayo Clin Proc 1991 Feb;66(2):155-59. PMID: 1899710.

70. Nigam A, Ahmed K, Drake-Lee AB. The value of preoperative estimation of haemoglobin in children undergoing tonsillectomy. Clin Otolaryngol Allied Sci 1990 Dec;15(6):549-51. PMID: 2073764.

71. O'Connor ME, Drasner K. Preoperative laboratory testing of children undergoing elective surgery. Anesth Analg. 1990 Feb;70(2):176-80.

72. Paterson KR, Caskie JP, Galloway DJ, et al. The pre-operative electrocardiogram: an assessment. Scott Med J. 1983 Apr;28(2):116-18. PMID: 6867689.

73. Perez A, Planell J, Bacardaz C, et al. Value of routine preoperative tests: a multicentre study in four general hospitals. Br J Anaesth. 1995 Mar;74(3):250-56. PMID: 7718366.

74. Pierre N, Moy LK, Redd S, et al. Evaluation of a pregnancy-testing protocol in adolescents undergoing surgery. J Pediatr Adolesc Gynecol. 1998 Aug;11(3):139-41. PMID: 9704304.

75. Roy WL, Lerman J, McIntyre BG. Is preoperative haemoglobin testing justified in children undergoing minor elective surgery? Can J Anaesth. 1991 Sep;38(6):700-03.

76. Sane SM, Worsing RA, Jr., Wiens CW, et al. Value of preoperative chest X-ray examinations in children. Pediatrics. 1977 Nov;60(5):669-72.

77. Silvestri L, Maffessanti M, Gregori D, et al. Usefulness of routine pre-operative chest radiography for anaesthetic management: a prospective multicentre pilot study. Eur J Anaesthesiol. 1999 Nov;16(11):749-60. PMID: 10713868.

78. Tape TG, Mushlin AI. How useful are routine chest x-rays of preoperative patients at risk for postoperative chest disease? J Gen Intern Med. 1988 Jan;3(1):15-20. PMID: 3339483.

79. Van Damme H, Pierard L, Gillain D, et al. Cardiac risk assessment before vascular surgery: a prospective study comparing clinical evaluation, dobutamine stress echocardiography, and dobutamine Tc-99m sestamibi tomoscintigraphy. Cardiovasc Surg. 1997 Feb;5(1):54-64. PMID: 9158124.

80. Leppo J, Plaja J, Gionet M, et al. Noninvasive evaluation of cardiac risk before elective vascular surgery. J Am Coll Cardiol. 1987 Feb;9(2):269-76. PMID: 3805515.

81. Phillips MB, Bendel RE, Crook JE, et al. Global health implications of preanesthesia medical examination for ophthalmic surgery. Anesthesiology. 2013;118(5):1038-45. PMID: 23508220.

82. Eagle KA, Berger PB, Calkins H, et al. ACC/AHA guideline update for perioperative cardiovascular evaluation for noncardiac surgery--executive summary: a report of the American College of Cardiology/American Heart Association Task Force on Practice Guidelines (Committee to Update the 1996 Guidelines on Perioperative Cardiovascular Evaluation for Noncardiac Surgery). J Am Coll Cardiol. 2002 Feb 6;39(3):542-53. PMID: 11823097.

83. Qaseem A, Snow V, Fitterman N, et al. Risk assessment for and strategies to reduce perioperative pulmonary complications for patients undergoing noncardiothoracic surgery: a guideline from the American College of Physicians. Ann Intern Med. 2006 Apr 18;144(8):575-80. PMID: 16618955.

84. Smetana GW, Lawrence VA, Cornell JE, et al. Preoperative pulmonary risk stratification for noncardiothoracic surgery: systematic review for the American College of Physicians. Ann Intern Med. 2006 Apr 18;144(8):581-95. PMID: 16618956.

85. Schein OD, Katz J, Bass EB, et al. The value of routine preoperative medical testing before cataract surgery. Study of Medical Testing for Cataract Surgery. N Engl J Med. 2000 Jan 20;342(3):168-75. PMID: 10639542.

86. Myers E, Sanders GD, Ravi D, et al. Evaluating the Potential Use of Modeling and Value-of-Information Analysis for Future Research Prioritization Within the Evidence-based Practice Center Program. (Prepared by the Duke Evidence-based Practice Center under Contract No. 290-2007-10066-I.) AHRQ Publication No. 11-EHC030-EF. Rockville, MD: Agency for Healthcare Research and Quality. June 2011. Available at: www.effectivehealthcare.ahrq.gov/reports/final.cfm.

Appendix A. Literature Search Strategy

July 22, 2013

Five databases searched:

Ovid MEDLINE(R) 1946 to July Week 3 2013

EBM Reviews - Cochrane Database of Systematic Reviews 2005 to July 2013

EBM Reviews - Cochrane Central Register of Controlled Trials to July 2013

EBM Reviews - Health Technology Assessment to 2nd Quarter 2013

Ovid Healthstar - 1966 to July 2013

#	Searches <<description>>	Results
1	exp "Ambulatory Surgical Procedures"/	21168
2	exp "Surgical Procedures Elective"/	16102
3	exp "Preoperative Care"/	105812
4	ambulatory surg*.af.	23281
5	elective surg*.af.	15691
6	(preop or pre-op or pre-operative or pre operative or preoperative or "pre operative").af.	334692
7	*or/1-6* <<*pre-op or surgery*>>	**389716**
8	"Diagnostic Tests Routine"/	13032
9	((diagnostic or laboratory) adj10 (test or tests or testing)).mp. [mp=ti, ab, ot, nm, hw, kf, ps, rs, ui, tx, kw, ct, sh]	151480
10	exp "Sensitivity & Specificity"/	705830
11	"Predictive Value of Tests"/	245895
12	exp Mass Screening/	215864
13	(sensitivit* or specificit* or predictive value* or accuracy or likelihood ratio* or screening or false negative*).mp. [mp=ti, ab, ot, nm, hw, kf, ps, rs, ui, tx, kw, ct, sh]	2551208
14	*or/8-13* <<*tests, general*>>	**2674572**
15	*(comment or editorial or letter or news).pt.* <<*exclusions*>> *(exclusions)*	**2167401**
16	Electrocardiography.af.	284718
17	(ecg or electrocardiogra*).mp. [mp=ti, ab, ot, nm, hw, kf, ps, rs, ui, tx, kw, ct, sh]	334122
18	*16 or 17* <<*ECG*>>	*334135*
19	Radiography/	38507
20	((chest or thoracic) and (xray* or x-ray* or radiograph* or roentgenography)).af.	168282
21	exp Radiography Thoracic/	52842
22	*19 or 20 or 21* <<*CXR*>>	*211507*
23	exp Hemoglobins/	146648
24	(hemoglobin* or haemoglobin*).mp. [mp=ti, ab, ot, nm, hw, kf, ps, rs, ui, tx, kw, ct, sh]	226734
25	exp Blood Cell Count/	171734
26	blood count.mp. [mp=ti, ab, ot, nm, hw, kf, ps, rs, ui, tx, kw, ct, sh]	7872
27	white blood cell count.mp. [mp=ti, ab, ot, nm, hw, kf, ps, rs, ui, tx, kw, ct, sh]	9979
28	leukocyte count.mp. [mp=ti, ab, ot, nm, hw, kf, ps, rs, ui, tx, kw, ct, sh]	74872
29	platelet count.mp. [mp=ti, ab, ot, nm, hw, kf, ps, rs, ui, tx, kw, ct, sh]	40843
30	*23 or 24 or 25 or 26 or 27 or 28 or 29* <<*blood counts*>>	*415342*
31	exp Hemostasis/ or exp Hemostasis, Surgical/	149861
32	exp Hematologic Tests/	299343
33	(h?emostasis or h?ematologic test*).mp.	62604
34	exp Blood Coagulation Tests/	48188
35	exp Blood Coagulation/	65371
36	blood coagulation/	45934
37	blood coagulation test.af.	48
38	blood examination.af.	1063
39	exp blood clotting test/	0
40	exp Partial Thromboplastin Time/	8076
41	exp International Normalized Ratio/	6118
42	(partial thromboplastin time or PTT).mp. [mp=ti, ab, ot, nm, hw, kf, ps, rs, ui, tx, kw, ct, sh]	16258
43	(international normali?ed ratio or INR).mp. [mp=ti, ab, ot, nm, hw, kf, ps, rs, ui, tx, kw, ct, sh]	13053
44	prothrombin time.mp. or exp Prothrombin Time/	20444
45	bleeding time.mp. or exp Bleeding Time/	7413
46	whole blood coagulation time.mp. or exp Whole Blood Coagulation Time/	1831
47	*or/31-46* <<*hemostasis*>>	*455996*

#	Searches <<description>>	Results
48	exp Biochemistry/	500169
49	biochemistry/	17835
50	blood chemistry.af.	4410
51	exp Blood Chemical Analysis/	162574
52	exp Glucose Tolerance Test/	41299
53	(glucose tolerance or glucose test*).mp.	63039
54	exp Diagnostic Techniques, Urological/	163541
55	diagnostic techniques urological.af.	887
56	exp Urinalysis/	7200
57	(urine analysis or urinalysis or dipstick).mp.	19061
58	exp Kidney Function Tests/	91577
59	kidney function test*/	0
60	((kidney function or renal function) adj10 test*).mp.	33772
61	exp Electrolytes/	568493
62	electrolyt*.mp.	111412
63	creatinine.mp. or exp Creatinine/	147554
64	blood urea nitrogen.mp. or exp blood urea nitrogen/	20558
65	urea nitrogen blood level.af.	91
66	*or/48-65* *<<laboratory tests>>*	*1562962*
67	blood glucose.mp. or exp blood glucose/	207294
68	blood sugar.mp.	12086
69	glucose test*.mp.	2139
70	glucose blood level.af.	1148
71	*or/67-70* *<<blood glucose>>*	*212625*
72	exp pregnancy tests/	4810
73	pregnancy test*.mp.	6490
74	exp chronic gonadotropin, beta subunit, human/ or beta hcg.mp.	4232
75	*or/72-74* *<<pregnancy test>>*	*10542*
76	exp hemoglobinopathies/	53186
77	h?emoglobinopath*.mp.	8204
78	exp Anemia, sickle cell/ or sickle cell.mp.	30193
79	*or/76-78* *<<sickle cell test>>*	*57996*
80	exp respiratory function tests/	323769
81	lung function test.af.	976
82	exp airway resistance/	18628
83	exp respiratory airflow/	62793
84	exp lung volume measurements/	48566
85	lung volume/	0
86	exp vital capacity/	34096
87	(vital capacity or VC).mp.	41126
88	exp forced expiratory flow rates/	16550
89	exp forced expiratory volume/	37389
90	forced expiratory volume/	37389
91	((pulmonary function or respiratory function or lung function) adj10 test*).mp.	75895
92	(forced expiratory volume or fev).mp.	54666
93	(peak expiratory flow rate or PEF).mp. or exp peak expiratory flow rate/	16902
94	forced respiratory function.af.	1
95	exp blood gas analysis/ or blood gas*.mp.	67174

#	Searches	<<description>>	Results
96	*or/80-95*	*<<pulmonary tests>>*	*363601*
97	**18 or 22 or 30 or 47 or 66 or 71 or 75 or 79 or 96**	**<<tests, specific>>**	**3102325**
98	**(and/7,14,97) not 15**	**<<pre-op & tests, general & tests, specific *not* exclusions>>**	**7985**
99	limit 98 to yr="1890 - 1999"		2622
100	remove duplicates from 99		1344
101	limit 98 to yr="2000 - 2013"		5363
102	remove duplicates from 101		2916
103	(preop$ and test$).ti	<<terms added after peer review>>	372
104	103 not (98 or 15)		262
105	**100 or 102**　　　　　　　　　**<<FINAL YIELD, deduplicated>>**		**4581**
	Ovid MEDLINE(R)		(4346)
	EBM Reviews - Cochrane Database of Systematic Reviews		(192)
	EBM Reviews - Cochrane Central Register of Controlled Trials		(12)
	EBM Reviews - Health Technology Assessment		(6)
	Ovid Healthstar		(25)

Appendix B. List of Rejected Articles

Author	Year	PMID	Rejection reason
Adams JG.	1992	1524480	Test not performed in all patients (only "ad hoc")
Akin BV.	1987	3565429	Not anesthesia-involved surgery or procedure
Allison JG.	1996	8712570	No outcome of interest
Ammar AD.	1996	8976360	Non-comparative and no process outcome (eg, LOS, surgical delay/cancel, follow-up testing, etc.)
Archer C.	1993	8269561	Not primary study
Arieta CE.	2004	15029333	Non-comparative and no process outcome (eg, LOS, surgical delay/cancel, follow-up testing, etc.)
Asimakopoulos G.	1998	9654879	Not test of interest
Bach DS.	1998	9792564	Not test of interest
Barazzoni F.	1999	10356863	No comparison of interest
Barazzoni F.	2002	12201191	No outcome of interest
Barisione G.	1997	9192933	Non-comparative and no process outcome (eg, LOS, surgical delay/cancel, follow-up testing, etc.)
Basora M.	2006	17105489	Not test of interest
Best WR.	2002	11893128	Test not performed in all patients (only "ad hoc")
Blery C.	1986	2867356	Non-comparative and no process outcome (eg, LOS, surgical delay/cancel, follow-up testing, etc.)
Bléry C.	1987	3578950	No comparison of interest
Boghosian SG.	1987	3805556	Non-comparative and no process outcome (eg, LOS, surgical delay/cancel, follow-up testing, etc.)
Boland BJ.	1995	7900740	Not anesthesia-involved surgery or procedure
Boothe P.	1995	7614645	Restricted to patients with 24 hour LOS
Brady AR.	2000	10848851	Test not performed in all patients (only "ad hoc")
Bryson GL.	2006	16527786	Test not performed in all patients (only "ad hoc")
Carliner NH.	1985	4014040	Non-comparative and no process outcome (eg, LOS, surgical delay/cancel, follow-up testing, etc.)
Catchlove BR.	1979	537560	Not primary study
Chalas E.	1992	1550175	Test not performed in all patients (only "ad hoc")
Cherng YG.	1998	10399512	Only analyze test results as predictor of/association with outcomes
Christian KW.	1988	3213942	No comparison of interest
Clelland C.	1996	8865786	Not test of interest
Close HL.	1994	7991252	Non-comparative and no process outcome (eg, LOS, surgical delay/cancel, follow-up testing, etc.)
Conway JB.	1992	1464132	Evaluation of ad hoc referral to preoperative clinic
Cooper JD.	2010	20672369	Not primary study
Crapo RO.	1986	3715720	Non-comparative and no process outcome (eg, LOS, surgical delay/cancel, follow-up testing, etc.)
Crawford MW.	2005	16326676	Test not performed in all patients (only "ad hoc")
De la Matta Martín M.	2011	21608275	No comparison of interest
de Vries TW.	1992	1407139	No comparison of interest
Deffarges C.	1990	2240691	Test not performed in all patients (only "ad hoc")
Delahunt B.	1980	6782527	Non-comparative and no process outcome (eg, LOS, surgical delay/cancel, follow-up testing, etc.)
Dzankic S.	2001	11473849	Non-comparative and no process outcome (eg, LOS, surgical delay/cancel, follow-up testing, etc.)
Eisenberg JM.	1982	7055424	No outcome of interest
Eisert S.	2006	17080336	Non-comparative and no process outcome (eg, LOS, surgical delay/cancel, follow-up testing, etc.)
Epstein AM.	1986	3960081	Not anesthesia-involved surgery or procedure

Author	Year	PMID	Rejection reason
Escolano F.	1994	8016434	No comparison of interest
Escolano F.	1996	9005498	No comparison of interest
Feely MA	2013	23547574	Not primary study
Fischer SP.	1996	8694365	No outcome of interest
Fischer SP.	1999	10331340	Not primary study
Fleisher LA.	1999	10512254	Test not performed in all patients (only "ad hoc")
Fok CS	2013	23219547	Non-comparative and no process outcome (eg, LOS, surgical delay/cancel, follow-up testing, etc.)
Fourcade RO.	1989	2624447	Non-comparative and no process outcome (eg, LOS, surgical delay/cancel, follow-up testing, etc.)
France FH.	1997	9489121	Not primary study
Gagner M.	1990	2383834	Test not performed in all patients (only "ad hoc")
García-Miguel FJ.	2002	11898449	Non-comparative and no process outcome (eg, LOS, surgical delay/cancel, follow-up testing, etc.)
García-Miguel FJ.	2002	12025252	Non-comparative and no process outcome (eg, LOS, surgical delay/cancel, follow-up testing, etc.)
Gauss A.	2001	11135720	Non-comparative and no process outcome (eg, LOS, surgical delay/cancel, follow-up testing, etc.)
Goldman L.	1977	904659	Non-comparative and no process outcome (eg, LOS, surgical delay/cancel, follow-up testing, etc.)
Hennrikus WL.	2001	11521041	No outcome of interest
Houry S.	1995	7793487	Analyses include history and physical examination also
Howells RC.	1997	9419090	Test not performed in all patients (only "ad hoc")
Huang CJ.	2006	16643221	Not test of interest
Hubbell FA.	1985	3965947	Not anesthesia-involved surgery or procedure
Hux J.	2003	14628523	Test not performed in all patients (only "ad hoc")
Ishaq M.	1997	9510631	Test not performed in all patients (only "ad hoc")
Jacobsen J.	1987	3826581	Not primary study
Jakobsson A.	1984	6143913	Not primary study
Jeavons SJ.	1987	2963612	Test not performed in all patients (only "ad hoc")
Jones MW.	1988	3408144	Not primary study
Kabakibi A.	1998	9535391	Test not performed in all patients (only "ad hoc")
Kerr IH.	1974	4621286	Not primary study
Kertai MD.	2003	12572926	Test not performed in all patients (only "ad hoc")
Kim SK.	1987	3269245	Test not performed in all patients (only "ad hoc")
Koscielny J.	2007	17694224	Diagnostic test; Non-comparative and no process outcome (eg, LOS, surgical delay/cancel, follow-up testing, etc.);Only analyze test results as predictor of/association with outcomes
Kozak EA.	1994	8082343	Not anesthesia-involved surgery or procedure
Kroenke K.	1986	3772598	Not anesthesia-involved surgery or procedure
Krupski WC.	2000	10737150	Test not performed in all patients (only "ad hoc")
Lamers RJ.	1989	2586653	No comparison of interest
Landesberg G.	1997	9357456	Not test of interest
Lawrence VA.	1989	2511275	Not primary study
Leppo J	1987	3805515	Not test of interest
Levy PA.	1979	10315061	No outcome of interest

Author	Year	PMID	Rejection reason
Lim EH.	2003	14620724	Test not performed in all patients (only "ad hoc")
Liu LL.	2002	12133011	Test not performed in all patients (only "ad hoc")
Macpherson DS.	1990	2240920	Test not performed in all patients (only "ad hoc")
Macpherson DS.	1993	8441296	Not primary study
Mamode N.	2001	11735198	Non-comparative and no process outcome (eg, LOS, surgical delay/cancel, follow-up testing, etc.)
McGirt MJ.	2006	16723885	Test not performed in all patients (only "ad hoc")
McKee RF.	1987	3631872	Non-comparative and no process outcome (eg, LOS, surgical delay/cancel, follow-up testing, etc.)
Mendelson DS.	1987	3659353	Test not performed in all patients (only "ad hoc")
Meyer RA.	1970	5266022	Non-comparative and no process outcome (eg, LOS, surgical delay/cancel, follow-up testing, etc.)
Michel C.	1989	2717842	No comparison of interest
Moorman JR.	1985	3929661	Not anesthesia-involved surgery or procedure
Morales-Orozco C.	2005	15888267	No comparison of interest
Morise AP.	1987	3565461	No data specific to routine tests, only to combined test and physical examination
Moyes LH	2013	23484995	Non-comparative and no process outcome (eg, LOS, surgical delay/cancel, follow-up testing, etc.)
Murdoch CJ.	1999	10460569	Test not performed in all patients (only "ad hoc")
Muskett AD.	1986	3774723	Test not performed in all patients (only "ad hoc")
Myers ER.	1994	8127539	Test not performed in all patients (only "ad hoc")
Nascimento MA.	2005	15905943	No comparison of interest
Nze PU.	2008	18686829	Non-comparative and no process outcome (eg, LOS, surgical delay/cancel, follow-up testing, etc.)
Ogunseyinde AO.	1988	2845755	No outcome of interest
Ohrlander T.	2012	22801403	Not test of interest
Older P	1993	8365279	Non-comparative and no process outcome (eg, LOS, surgical delay/cancel, follow-up testing, etc.)
Older P.	1999	10453862	Not test of interest
Pal KM.	1998	10323056	Test not performed in all patients (only "ad hoc")
Papaceit J.	2003	14599421	No comparison of interest
Parolari A.	2012	22269725	Test not performed in all patients (only "ad hoc")
Patel RI.	1992	1632540	Test not performed in all patients (only "ad hoc")
Perlíková I.	1994	8052921	Not test of interest
Poe RH.	1988	3122567	Only analyze test results as predictor of/association with outcomes
Poldermans D.	1993	8491005	Not test of interest
Poldermans D	2006	16949487	No outcomes of interest
Pollard JB.	1996	8694327	Test not performed in all patients (only "ad hoc")
Prause G.	1994	8179172	No comparison of interest
Qaseem A.	2006	16618955	Not primary study
Rabkin SW.	1979	111793	Mix of elective and emergency surgery; no outcomes of interest
Rabkin SW.	1983	6848157	Test not performed in all patients (only "ad hoc")
Rader ES.	1978	76362	Non-comparative and no process outcome (eg, LOS, surgical delay/cancel, follow-up testing, etc.)
Rajamanickam A.	2007	18368871	Not primary study
Ritz JP.	1997	9574329	No comparison of interest

B-4

Author	Year	PMID	Rejection reason
Robbins JA.	1979	529881	Not primary study
Roux A.	1993	8432567	Emergency surgery (trauma)
Royal College of Radiologists	1979	87976	Test not performed in all patients (only "ad hoc")
Rucker L.	1983	6645012	Not anesthesia-involved surgery or procedure
Rutten CL.	1995	7777084	No comparison of interest
Sagel SS.	1974	4413189	Not anesthesia-involved surgery or procedure
Samková A.	2012	21967473	Analysis only of abnormal test results (in outpatient hematology clinic)
Sanders DP.	1989	2511563	Test not performed in all patients (only "ad hoc")
Sandler G.	1979	466256	Not anesthesia-involved surgery or procedure
Savina MD.	1986	3720934	Non-comparative and no process outcome (eg, LOS, surgical delay/cancel, follow-up testing, etc.)
Scheckenbach K.	2008	17581692	Non-comparative and no process outcome (eg, LOS, surgical delay/cancel, follow-up testing, etc.)
Schmidt JL.	1990	2228707	Not primary study
Schwaab M.	2008	17963191	No comparison of interest
Schwaab M.	2009	19034824	No comparison of interest
Seymour DG.	1983	6869118	Non-comparative and no process outcome (eg, LOS, surgical delay/cancel, follow-up testing, etc.)
Seymour DG.	1982	7170281	Non-comparative and no process outcome (eg, LOS, surgical delay/cancel, follow-up testing, etc.)
Shafritz R.	1997	9293826	Not test of interest
Smetana GW.	2006	16618956	Not primary study
Sommerville TE.	1992	1738905	Test not performed in all patients (only "ad hoc")
Starsnic MA.	1997	9195353	Did not report outcome of interest by group (or excluding elective testing)
Steib A.	1994	7826793	Non-comparative and no process outcome (eg, LOS, surgical delay/cancel, follow-up testing, etc.)
Stevens RD.	2004	15460545	Not primary study
Suchman AL.	1986	3723774	Test not performed in all patients (only "ad hoc")
Syed MA.	1998	9732881	Not anesthesia-involved surgery or procedure
Tait AR.	1997	9327318	Test not performed in all patients (only "ad hoc")
Tallo FS.	2007	17906760	No comparison of interest
Thanh NX.	2010	20054679	Not clearly "routine"; No outcomes of interest
Thompson RE.	1979	121382	Not primary study
Tisi GM.	1979	373529	Not primary study
Tomita M.	2010	21069496	Test not performed in all patients (only "ad hoc")
Troisi N.	2010	20472385	Non-comparative and no process outcome (eg, LOS, surgical delay/cancel, follow-up testing, etc.)
Turnbull JM.	1987	3592875	Test not performed in all patients (only "ad hoc")
Twersky RS.	1996	8694346	Not primary study
Vogt AW.	1997	9278827	Test not performed in all patients (only "ad hoc")
Wattsman TA.	1997	8985077	Test not performed in all patients (only "ad hoc")
Weksler N.	2003	12770652	Study comparing surgery postponement due to high BP vs. none
Wiencek RG.	1987	3605857	No PDF could be retrieve
Williams GD.	1999	10468251	Non-comparative and no process outcome (eg, LOS, surgical delay/cancel, follow-up testing, etc.)

Author	Year	PMID	Rejection reason
Wilson J.	1999	10213716	Not test of interest
Wilson ME.	1980	7370563	Survey of anesthesiologists, essentially
Wilson RF.	1979	435059	Not anesthesia-involved surgery or procedure
Wood RA.	1981	7254966	Test not performed in all patients (only "ad hoc")
Yipintsoi T.	1989	2723562	Too unclear a linkage between ECG results and subsequent management

Appendix C. Summary Tables

Table C-1. Study characteristics

Author, Year PMID Country	Design Funding	Year of Study Start Study Duration	Inclusion	Exclusion	Surgery setting Population	Type of anesthesia	Who order the tests	Surgical procedure	Severity of surgery grades
Comparative studies									
Almanaseer, 2005 15528897 US	Retrospective NRS Foundation: Blue Cross Blue Shield of Michigan Foundation	1994 7 mo	Patients seen in the Preoperative Clinic before scheduled noncardiac surgery	Urgent or emergent surgery	Hospital Adults	NR	Other (Hospital physician in General Internal Medicine Preoperative Clinic)	General/ Various	Grade 1-4
Cavallini, 2004 15506597 Italy	RCT NR	2002 13 mo	Admitted to day surgery for elective cataract surgery under local anesthesia	Ongoing treatment with anticoagulants or subcutaneous insulin therapy	Day surgery unit Adults	Local	Primary care physician, Other (health care personnel)	Cataract	Grade 1

Author, Year PMID Country	Design Funding	Year of Study Start Study Duration	Inclusion	Exclusion	Surgery setting Population	Type of anesthesia	Who order the tests	Surgical procedure	Severity of surgery grades
Chung 2009 19151274 Canada	RCT Professional organization	2008 nd	Patients scheduled to undergoing orthopedic, plastic, general, urology, ophthalmologic (excluding cataract), or spinal surgery who were >16 yo and were scheduled to be discharged home on the same day.	Undergoing ambulatory cardiovascular, thoracic, neurosurgical or cataract surgery, or any of the following medical conditions: i) MI within 3 mo, previous heart surgery or angioplasty; ii) angina, Canadian Cardiovascular Class (CCS) 3, angina on walking 1 flight of stair or two blocks; CCS 4, angina with activities of daily living, including at rest; iii) dyspnea, CCS 3 shortness of breath 1 flight of stairs or two blocks, CCS 4 shortness of breath with activities of daily living, including at rest; iv) arrhythmias; v) history of coagulopathy or blood disorder; vi) history of significant anemia; vii) history of significant liver disease; viii) history of significant renal	Hospital Adults	General, Local, Neuraxial block, Sedation/MAC only	Surgeon	General/ Various	Grade 2-4

C-3

Author, Year PMID Country	Design Funding	Year of Study Start Study Duration	Inclusion	Exclusion	Surgery setting Population	Type of anesthesia	Who order the tests	Surgical procedure	Severity of surgery grades
Falcone 2003 14689407 US	RCT The Mid-Atlantic Affiliate American Heart Association, Grant-in-Aid.	1997 12 mo	Patients undergoing elective abdominal aortic, infrainguinal, and carotid vascular surgery.	A prior complete cardiac evaluation by their primary physician or cardiologist, cardiac revascularization within 1 year, or, in only a few, because of refusal to enroll.	Hospital Adults	NR	NR	Vascular	NR
Finegan, 2005 15983141 Canada	Prospective NRS Hospital	NA 17 wk	All patients attending the clinic who were admitted to hospital following their procedure, (including those referred subsequently for subspecialty consultation by internal medicine and cardiology) were enrolled prospectively in the study.	those scheduled for cardiac surgery or undergoing dialysis at the time of the clinic visit	Hospital Adults	NR	Surgeon, Anesthesiologist	General/ Various	Grade 1- 4

Author, Year PMID Country	Design Funding	Year of Study Start Study Duration	Inclusion	Exclusion	Surgery setting Population	Type of anesthesia	Who order the tests	Surgical procedure	Severity of surgery grades
Larocque, 1994 7922901 Canada	Retrospective NRS NR	NA NA	Underwent cataract surgery, TURP, laparoscopic cholecystectomy, hip arthroplasty, abdominal hysterectomy, breast reduction, radical neck dissection, any cardiovascular surgery, any thoracic surgery	NR	Hospital Adults	General, Local, Nerve block, Neuraxial block	NR	General/ Various	Grade 1-4
Leonard, 1975 1095116 UK	RCT (two trials running simultaneously) NR	1973 39 wk	All children admitted to the hospital who were surgical patients expected to stay in hospital <1 week.	Day cases and those admitted directly to two surgical wards	Hospital Pediatric	NR	NR	General/ Various	NR
Lira, 2001 11558245 Brazil	RCT Hospital	2000 11 mo	Scheduled to undergo cataract surgery	<40 yo; undergoing surgery on the second eye; were to receive general anesthesia; had had MI within the preceding 3 months.	Hospital Adults	NR	Physician	Cataract	Grade 1

Author, Year PMID Country	Design Funding	Year of Study Start / Study Duration	Inclusion	Exclusion	Surgery setting / Population	Type of anesthesia	Who order the tests	Surgical procedure	Severity of surgery grades
Mancuso 1999 10203622 US	Retrospective NRS Hospital	1991 4 y, 5 mo	All orthopedic patients undergoing ambulatory surgery who were referred to a single medical consultant (the author) during the 2 years before and the 2 years after the new guidelines	NR	Ambulatory/outpatient clinic Adults & Pediatrics	General, Local, Nerve block, Neuraxial block	Surgeon	Orthopedic	NR
Meneghini, 1998 9483592 Italy	Retrospective NRS NR	1981 15 y	All children ASA physical status 1 and 2 who underwent an elective minor surgical procedure in the last 15 years.	Former preterm infants of less than 60 weeks postconceptual ages.	NR Pediatric	General, Local, Nerve block, Neuraxial block (epidural, spinal), Sedation/ MAC only	NR	General/ Various	Grade 1
Mignonsin, 1996 8762245 Ivory Coast	Pro- and retrospective NRS NR	NR 12 mo	ASA I-III, undergoing elective surgery (gastrointestinal, trauma/ orthopedic, urology, gynecology)	Urgent surgery, major surgery (neurosurgery, thoracic surgery)	Hospital Adults & Pediatrics	NR	NR	General/ Various	Grade 2 & 3

Author, Year PMID Country	Design Funding	Year of Study Start / Study Duration	Inclusion	Exclusion	Surgery setting / Population	Type of anesthesia	Who order the tests	Surgical procedure	Severity of surgery grades
Schein, 2000 10639542 US	RCT / Government	1995 / NA	Scheduled to undergo cataract surgery in a single eye	<50 yo, were to receive general anesthesia, had a myocardial infarction within the preceding 3 months, had undergone any preoperative medical testing during the 28 days before enrollment, or could not speak English or Spanish.	A mix of private practices, academic medical centers, and community hospitals. / Adults	Local	Other ("Health care provider")	Cataract	Grade 1
Wyatt, 1989 2729769 US	Retrospective NRS / NR	1985 / 12 mo	Patients undergoing ambulatory surgery and scheduled to receive anesthesia	Scheduled to receive straight local anesthesia administrated by surgeon	Ambulatory/outpatient clinic / Adults	General, Local, Nerve block, Neuraxial block	NR	General/ Various	NR
Zwack, 1997 9051441 US	Retrospective NRS / NR	NA / 6 y	Patients scheduled for tonsillectomy, adenoidectomy, or adenotonsillectomy at a children's hospital	NR	Hospital / Pediatric	NR	Surgeon	Tonsillectomy	Grade 2

Single arm studies

Author, Year PMID Country	Design Funding	Year of Study Start Study Duration	Inclusion	Exclusion	Surgery setting Population	Type of anesthesia	Who order the tests	Surgical procedure	Severity of surgery grades
Aghajanian, 1991 1923209 US	Retrospective cohort NR	1990 6 mo	Patients scheduled for elective gynecologic operations	Emergency cases	Hospital Adults	NR	NR	General/ Various	Grade 2,3
Alsumait, 2002 12116695 Kuwait	Prospective Cohort NR	1999 8 mo	General surgical cases (elective and emergency)	NR	Hospital Adults & Pediatric	NR	NR	General/ Various	NR
Azzam, 1996 8712424 US	Retrospective cohort NR	1992 2 y	Postmenarchal patients presenting for surgery and anesthesia at the freestanding pediatric hospital service.	NR	Hospital Pediatric	NR	Other (nurses)	General/ Various	NR
Baron, 1992 1470961 US	Retrospective cohort NR	NA NA	All patients 18 yo and younger in the 'same day surgery' log books scheduled for elective operations	Known sickle cell disease or other hematologic conditions	Hospital Pediatric	NR	NR	General/ Various	Grade 1-3

C-8

Author, Year PMID Country	Design / Funding	Year of Study Start / Study Duration	Inclusion	Exclusion	Surgery setting / Population	Type of anesthesia	Who order the tests	Surgical procedure	Severity of surgery grades
Bhuripanyo, 1990 2345323 Thailand	Retrospective cohort / NR	1987 / 7 mo	Patient's age ≥15 yo who attend outpatients clinics of the department of Obstetrics and Gynecology, Orthopedics, Eye and Otolaryngology who were scheduled for an elective operation	Not admitted for operation from outpatient department. Scheduled for cardiothoracic operations. Missing CXR.	Hospital / Adults & Pediatric	NR	NR	General/Various	NR
Bhuripanyo, 1992 1293256 Thailand	Prospective cohort / NR	NA / NA	>40 yo; patients who attended the outpatient clinics of the departments of surgery, ob-gyn, orthopedics, eye, or ENT and were scheduled for elective operation	Patients scheduled for cardiothoracic operations	Hospital / Adults	NR	NR	General/Various	NR

Author, Year PMID Country	Design Funding	Year of Study Start Study Duration	Inclusion	Exclusion	Surgery setting Population	Type of anesthesia	Who order the tests	Surgical procedure	Severity of surgery grades
Bhuripanyo, 1995 7622976 Thailand	Prospective cohort NR	1987 NA	Patient's age ≥15 yo who attend outpatients clinics of the department of Obstetrics and Gynecology, Orthopedics, Eye and Otolaryngology who were scheduled for an elective operation	Missing CBC. No surgery due to underlying disease or nonmedical reasons	Ambulatory/ outpatient clinic Adults & Pediatric	NR	NR	General/ Various	NR
Bhuripanyo, 1995 7629451 Thailand	Prospective cohort NR	1987 7 mo	Patients ≥15yo who attend the outpatients clinics of the department of Surgery, Obstetrics & Gynaecology, Orthopedics, Eye and Otolaryngology and were scheduled for elective operation.	Not admitted for operation from outpatient clinic, scheduled for genitourinary tract operation, missing urinalysis.	Ambulatory/outpatient clinic Adults & Pediatric	NR	NR	General/ Various	NR

Author, Year PMID Country	Design Funding	Year of Study Start Study Duration	Inclusion	Exclusion	Surgery setting Population	Type of anesthesia	Who order the tests	Surgical procedure	Severity of surgery grades
Bouillot, 1996 8891616 France	Prospective cohort NR	1985 3 y	≥15 yo, undergoing a general or gastrointestinal operation under general, regional or local anesthesia	Surgery for carcinoma or thoracotomy	Hospital Adults & Pediatric	General, Local, Nerve block, Neuraxial block	Surgeon, Anesthesiologist	General/ Various	NR
Burk, 1992 1557263 US	Prospective cohort NR	NA 18 mo	Children undergoing tonsillectomy with or without adenoidectomy	NR	Hospital Pediatric	NR	NR	Tonsillectomy	Grade 2
Bushick, 1989 2585157 US	Retrospective cohort John Hartford Foundation	1984 12 mo	Patients admitted for elective orthopedic surgery with ASA level I or II in their preoperative anesthesia evaluation.	Missing laboratory data	Hospital Adults	NR	NR	Orthopedic	NR

C-11

Author, Year PMID Country	Design Funding	Year of Study Start / Study Duration	Inclusion	Exclusion	Surgery setting / Population	Type of anesthesia	Who order the tests	Surgical procedure	Severity of surgery grades
Carliner, 1986 3719447 US	Prospective cohort / Hospital and Veterans Administration	NA / NR	>40 yo who were scheduled to undergo elective thoracic, abdominal, or vascular surgery under general anesthesia. The patients had to have no contraindication to exercise testing and be willing to perform a preoperative exercise test.	Documented MI within the preceding 6 mo, unstable angina pectoris, congestive heart failure accompanied by increased jugular venous pressure or a ventricular gallop sound, hemodynamically significant aortic stenosis, Lown grades 4A or 4B ventricular arrhythmias at rest and controlled hypertension (systolic >=150 mmHg and diastolic >=110mm Hg)	Hospital / Adults	General	NR	General/ Various	NR
Charpak, 1988 3339918 France	Prospective cohort / Government	1983 / ~12 mo	Patients having operation or investigations under general or regional anesthesia	NR	Hospital / Adults & Pediatric	General, Nerve block, Neuraxial block	Surgeon, Anesthesiologist	General/ Various	Grade 1-4
Charpak, 1988 3383317 France	Prospective cohort / NR	1983 / 1 y	All surgery under general or regional anesthesia	Patients going to surgery under local anesthesia	Hospital / Adults	General, Neuraxial block	Surgeon, Anesthesiologist, Primary care physician, Other (residents)	General/ Various	Grade 1-4

Author, Year PMID Country	Design Funding	Year of Study Start / Study Duration	Inclusion	Exclusion	Surgery setting / Population	Type of anesthesia	Who order the tests	Surgical procedure	Severity of surgery grades
Correll, 2009 19417620 US	Retrospective cohort / Hospital	2003 / 2 mo	Elective surgical patients >50 y seen in a center for preoperative evaluation	NR	Hospital / Adults	NR	Other (Preoperative evaluation center)	General/Various	NR
Gabriel, 2000 10960200 France	Prospective cohort / NR	1996 / 1 y	Scheduled for tonsillectomy, inpatient or outpatient	NR	Hospital (outpatient or inpatient) / Pediatric	NR	NR	Tonsillectomy	Grade 2
Gold, 1992 1739358 US	Retrospective cohort / NR	NA / 15 mo	≥40 yo, scheduled for ambulatory surgery with general, regional or monitored anesthesia care	Local anesthesia only (without an anesthesiologist in attendance)	Hospital / Adults	General, Nerve block, Neuraxial block, Sedation/MAC only	NR	General/Various	Grade 1-3
Golub, 1992 1595835 US	Retrospective cohort / NR	1988 / 10 wk	Patients scheduled for ambulatory surgery	NR	Ambulatory/outpatient clinic / Adults	General, Local	NR	General/Various	NR
Haug, 1999 9915390 US	Prospective cohort / NR	1994 / 9 mo	All patients requiring general anesthesia or intravenous sedation for oral or maxillofacial surgery	NR	Office / Adults & Pediatric	General, Sedation/MAC only	NR	Head&neck/ENT	NR
Hoare, 1993 8289005 UK	Prospective cohort / NR	NA / 12 mo	All children admitted for ENT surgical procedures	Procedures for insertion of grommets	Hospital / Pediatric	NR	NR	Head&neck/ENT	Grade 1,2

Author, Year PMID Country	Design Funding	Year of Study Start Study Duration	Inclusion	Exclusion	Surgery setting Population	Type of anesthesia	Who order the tests	Surgical procedure	Severity of surgery grades
Ipp, 2011 21926874 US	Retrospective cohort NR	2000 7 y	12-18 yo with idiopathic scoliosis (AIS) presenting for spine surgery	Neuromuscular scoliosis, known cardiac disease, connective tissue disease, such as Marfan or Ehlers-Danlos syndrome, and any patient who presented with symptoms indicative of cardiac disease such as dyspnea, syncope, or pathologic murmur audible at the presurgical clearance examination	Hospital Pediatric	NR	Primary care physician	Orthopedic	Grade 3
Johnson, 1988 3175862 US	Prospective cohort NR	NA NR	Patients undergoing a variety of ambulatory surgical procedures	NR	NR Adults	General, Local, Sedation/ MAC only	Other (Physician's assistant)	General/ Various	NR
Johnson, 2002 12190758 UK	Prospective cohort NR	NA NR	Elective surgical patients	NR	Hospital Adults	NR	Surgeon	General/ Various	NR

Author, Year PMID Country	Design Funding	Year of Study Start / Study Duration	Inclusion	Exclusion	Surgery setting / Population	Type of anesthesia	Who order the tests	Surgical procedure	Severity of surgery grades
Kahn, 2008 18349183 US	Retrospective cohort NR	2005 1 y	Women of childbearing age (defined as the age between initial reported menses, and 1 y after last reported menses)	NR	Hospital Adults & Pediatric	NR	NR	General/ Various	NR
Kaplan, 1985 3999339 US	Retrospective cohort Government	1980 4 mo	Patients undergoing elective surgery	No matching coded discharge data (~2%)	Hospital Adults	NR	NR	General/ Various	NR
Lafferty, 2001 11528304 US	Prospective cohort NR	1998 3 mo	Undergoing electroconvulsive therapy (ECT)	NR	NR Adults	NR	NR	ECT	NR
Lawrence, 1988 3377621 US	Retrospective cohort NR	1984 12 mo	Patients undergoing elective knee procedure	<15 yo; procedures involving prostheses or those related to acute trauma	Hospital Adults & Pediatric	General, Neuraxial block	Other ("Physicians")	Orthopedic	Grade 2
Mallick, 2006 17143358 Saudi Arabia	Retrospective cohort NR	2004 1 y	Routine elective minor surgery procedures in the division of pediatric surgery	Any other active or ongoing diseases on admission, or medications that reflected active medical disease, which could influence the outcome of surgery, such as steroids	Hospital Pediatric	NR	NR	General/ Various	NR

Author, Year PMID Country	Design Funding	Year of Study Start Study Duration	Inclusion	Exclusion	Surgery setting Population	Type of anesthesia	Who order the tests	Surgical procedure	Severity of surgery grades
Malviya, 1996 8831334 US	Prospective cohort NR	1993 27 mo	All adolescent (<18 yo), postmenarchal female patients presenting for elective outpatient surgery	NR	Ambulatory/ outpatient clinic Pediatric	NR	NR	General/ Various	NR
Manning, 1987 3679679 US	Retrospective cohort NR	1983 18 mo	Patients scheduled for tonsillectomy, adenoidectomy or tonsillectomy with adenoidectomy	NR	Hospital Pediatric	NR	NR	Tonsillectomy	Grade 2
Mantha, 2005 15721730 India	Prospective cohort Professional organization (anesthesia)	NA NA	Adult patients scheduled for elective neurosurgery (intracranial, spinal, and peripheral neural procedures) during general anesthesia maintained by a single anesthesiologist	Required emergency intervention before surgery, had altered sensorium, or if they were bedridden before admission to the hospital	Hospital Adults	General	NR	Neurosurgery	Grade 4

Author, Year PMID Country	Design Funding	Year of Study Start Study Duration	Inclusion	Exclusion	Surgery setting Population	Type of anesthesia	Who order the tests	Surgical procedure	Severity of surgery grades
Narr, 1991 1899710 US	Retrospective cohort NR	1988 1 y	Elective surgery, healthy or have uncomplicated disease	Major cardiovascular disease, bleeding diathesis, severe pulmonary disease, uncontrolled diabetes mellitus, uncontrolled hypertension, renal disease, hepatitis, jaundice, or substance abuse and is ineligible for a preanesthetic examination but receives more extensive general medical evaluation. Also, patients who came to the Mayo Clinic for general medical examination and later had an operation as a result of that assessment.	Hospital Adults & Pediatric	NR	Primary care physician, Other (Other nonsurgical physician)	General/ Various	NR
Nigam, 1990 2073764 UK	Prospective cohort NR	NA 6 mo	Children admitted for tonsillectomy or tonsillectomy and adenoidectomy	NR	Hospital Pediatric	NR	NR	Tonsillectomy	Grade 2

Author, Year PMID Country	Design Funding	Year of Study Start Study Duration	Inclusion	Exclusion	Surgery setting Population	Type of anesthesia	Who order the tests	Surgical procedure	Severity of surgery grades
O'Connor, 1990 2301750 US	Retrospective cohort NR	1984 36 mo	<18 yo having a nonobstetric elective surgical procedure, general or spinal anesthesia	NR	Hospital Pediatric	General, Neuraxial block	NR	General/ Various	Grade 1, 3
Paterson, 1983 6867689 UK	Prospective cohort NR	NR NR	Admitted for elective surgery	NR	Hospital Adults & Pediatric	General	NR	General/ Various	Grade 1-3
Perez, 1995 7718366 Spain	Retrospective cohort Government	1990 1 y	Elective surgery and only routine preoperative tests were indicated	Emergency operations, patients with an ASA classification >II and those given local anesthesia without sedation	Hospital Adults & Pediatric	General, Nerve block, Neuraxial block	NR	General/ Various	NR
Pierre, 1998 9704304 US	Retrospective cohort Government	1994 21 mo	All females 12-21 yo presenting to the day surgery unit	NR	Ambulatory/outpatient clinic Pediatric	NR	NR	General/ Various	NR
Phillips, 2013 23508220 US	Prospective cohort Mayo Clinic	2009 2 y	All ophthalmic surgery patients were eligible and procedure types included cataract, oculoplastic, glaucoma, and retinal surgery	NR	Ambulatory/outpatient clinic Adults	NR	NR	Cataract	Grade 1

Author, Year PMID Country	Design Funding	Year of Study Start Study Duration	Inclusion	Exclusion	Surgery setting Population	Type of anesthesia	Who order the tests	Surgical procedure	Severity of surgery grades
Roy, 1991 1914052 Canada	Retrospective cohort NR	NA 4 mo	Children 1 month to 18 yo; ASA I or II; admitted to ambulatory care center for minor surgery	Children who scheduled for bone marrow biopsy, lumbar puncture and cystoscopy; children under chemotherapy, whose preoperative blood testing was undertaken at another laboratory and those who required sickle cell testing	Ambulatory/outpatient clinic Pediatric	General	NR	General/ Various	Grade 1,2
Sane, 1977 917629 US	Prospective cohort NR	1974 7 mo	Newborn to 19 yo who had preoperative chest roentgenograms in frontal and lateral views (all children undergoing general anesthesia receive a routine preoperative CXR)	NR	NR Pediatric	General	NR	General/ Various	NR

Author, Year PMID Country	Design Funding	Year of Study Start Study Duration	Inclusion	Exclusion	Surgery setting Population	Type of anesthesia	Who order the tests	Surgical procedure	Severity of surgery grades
Silvestri, 1999 10713868 Italy	Prospective cohort NR	1996 5 mo	Scheduled for elective surgery, met criteria for a preoperative CXR (protocol not described)	Underwent "selective" PCOR as a result of the pre-anesthetic examination	Hospital Adults & Pediatric	General, Local, Nerve block, Neuraxial block, Sedation/ MAC only	Surgeon	General/ Various	Grade 1-3
Tape, 1988 3339483 US	Retrospective cohort NR	1984 ~2 y	Adult patients admitted for vascular surgical procedures: abdominal aortic aneurysm repair, any type of vascular bypass procedure of the iliac, femoral, or popliteal arteries	Procedure was done emergently or vascular surgery was not the first surgical procedure of the hospital admission.	Hospital Adults	NR	NR	Vascular	Grade 3, 4
Van Damme, 1997 9158124 Belgium	Prospective cohort NR	1994 6 mo	Scheduled for elective major vascular surgery.	NR	Hospital Adults	NR	NR	Vascular	Grade 4

Abbreviations: ASA, American Surgical Association; CXR, chest x-ray; MAC, monitored anesthesia care; MI, myocardial infarction; mo, month; NA, not applicable; NR, not reported; NRS, nonrandomized (comparative) study; RCT, randomized controlled trial; UK, United Kingdom; US, United States; wk, week; y, year; yo, years old

Table C-2. Comparative studies: Baseline characteristics

Author Year PMID	Arm	Age, Mean (Range)	Male, %	Race	ASA	Diabetes	CHD/CAD/CHF	Stroke/TIA	Arrhythmia	HTN	Obesity	COPD	Asthma	CKD
Almamseer 2005 15528897	Per protocol	66 (24-92)	56	NR	NR	21% (NS between groups)	38% Angina, 18% Prior MI, 12% Prior bypass	NR	7% AFib	54%	NR	NR	NR	NR
	Elective	65 (22-93)	48	NR	NR	18%	26% Angina (P=0.002*), 25% Prior MI (P=0.03), 15% Prior bypass (NS)	NR	6% AFib (NS)	44 (P= 0.008)	NR	NR	NR	NR
Cavallini 2004 15506597	With preop testing	NR	NR	NR	NR	NR	NR	NR	NR	NR	NR	NR	NR	NR
	Without preop testing	NR	NR	NR	NR	NR	NR	NR	NR	NR	NR	NR	NR	NR
Chung 2009 19151274	Per protocol	16-39: 14%; 40-59: 51%; ≥60: 35%	58	NR	1-3	15%	5%	NR	1%	32%	NR	7% COPD or asthma	NR	1%
	No testing	16-39: 14%; 40-59: 51%; ≥60: 35%	58	NR	1-3	16%	5%	NR	1%	38%	NR	8% COPD or asthma	NR	0.2%
Falcone 2003 14689407	Routine	66 ± 10	65	W 91	NR	17	Prior CHF 2	NR	NR	65	NR	NR	NR	NR
	No testing	66 ± 11	70	W 81	NR	34	Prior CHF 4	NR	NR	75	NR	NR	NR	NR
Finegan 2005 15983141	Routine	57 ± 16	47	NR	1-4	NR	NR	NR	NR	NR	NR	NR	NR	NR
	Ad hoc	58 ± 16	49	NR	1-4	NR	NR	NR	NR	NR	NR	NR	NR	NR
Larocque 1994 7922901	Per protocol	59	40	NR	1-5	NR	36%	NR	NR	NR	NR	NR	NR	0.4%

C-21

Author Year PMID	Arm	Age, Mean (Range)	Male, %	Race	ASA	Diabetes	CHD/CAD/CHF	Stroke/TIA	Arrhythmia	HTN	Obesity	COPD	Asthma	CKD
	Ad hoc	60	40	NR	1-5	NR	37%	NR	NR	NR	NR	NR	NR	1%
Leonard 1975 1095116	Routine	<18y (implied)	64	NR	NR	NR	NR	NR	NR	NR	NR	NR	NR	NR
	Per protocol	<18y (implied)	NR	NR	NR	NR	NR	NR	NR	NR	NR	NR	NR	NR
Lira 2001 11558245	Routine	66 ± 12	55	NR	1- 3	19%	5%	1%	5%	49%	NR	6%	NR	2%
	Per protocol	67 ± 11	53	NR	1- 3	20%	4%	1%	4%	48%	NR	5%	NR	2%
Mancuso 1999 10203622	Routine	46 (16-82)	50	NR	Nr	3%	3%	NR	NR	13%	NR	"Pulmonary disease" 7%	NR	NR
	Per protocol	47 (17-86)	52	NR	NR	1%	1%	NR	NR	9%	NR	"Pulmonary disease" 8%	NR	NR
Meneghini 1998 9483592	Routine	4 (28d-16yo)	NR	NR	1, 2	NR	NR	NR	NR	NR	NR	NR	NR	NR
	Per protocol	3 (15d-17yo)	NR	NR	1, 2	NR	NR	NR	NR	NR	NR	NR	NR	NR
Mignonsin, 1996 8762245	Routine	38 (3-88)	61	Nr	1-3	NR	NR	NR	NR	NR	NR	NR	NR	NR
	Per protocol	41 (4-88)	72	NR	1	NR	NR	NR	NR	NR	NR	NR	NR	NR
Schein 2000 10639542	Routine	73 ± 8	39	W 81%; B 6%, H 1%, Oth 2%	1-4	15%	4% CHF, 14% MI or prior CABG	8%	16%	47%	NR	14% COPD or asthma	NR	2.9% "Renal disease"
	No testing	74 ± 8	40	W 81%; B 6%, H 1%, Oth 2%	1-4	15%	4% CHF, 14% MI or prior CABG	9%	17%	47%	NR	14% COPD or asthma	NR	2.8% "Renal disease"
Wyatt 1989 2729769	Per protocol	NR	NR	NR	NR	NR	NR	NR	NR	NR	NR	NR	NR	NR
	Elective	NR	NR	NR	NR	NR	NR	NR	NR	NR	NR	NR	NR	NR

Author Year PMID	Arm	Age, Mean (Range)	Male, %	Race	ASA	Diabetes	CHD/CAD/CHF	Stroke/ TIA	Arrhythmia	HTN	Obesity	COPD	Asthma	CKD
Zwack 1997 9051441	Routine	(~2-17)	NR	NR	NR	NR	NR	NR	NR	NR	NR	NR	NR	NR
	Per protocol	(~2-17)	NR	NR	NR	NR	NR	NR	NR	NR	NR	NR	NR	NR

Abbreviations: AFib, atrial fibrillation or flutter; ASA, American Surgical Association category; B, black; CABG, coronary artery bypass grafting; CAD, coronary artery disease; CHD, coronary heart disease; CHF, coronary heart failure; CKD, chronic kidney disease; COPD, chronic obstructive pulmonary disease; H, Hispanic; HTN, hypertension; MI, myocardial infarction; NR, not reported; NS, nonsignificant; Oth, other race; preop, preoperative; TIA, transient ischemic attack; W, white.
* P value between groups.

Table C-3. Noncomparative studies: Baseline characteristics

Author Year PMID	Arm	Age, y Mean (Range)	Male, %	Race	ASA	Diabetes	CHD/CAD/CHF	Stroke/TIA	Arrhythmia	HTN	Obesity	COPD	Asthma	CKD
Aghajanian 1991 1923209	Routine	NR	0	NR	NR	NR	NR	NR	NR	NR	NR	NR	NR	NR
Alsumait 2002 12116695	Routine	Range 12-90	NR	NR	NR	NR	NR	NR	NR	NR	NR	NR	NR	NR
Azzam 1996 8712424	Routine	15 (11-20)	0	NR	NR	NR	NR	NR	NR	NR	NR	NR	NR	NR
Baron 1992 1470961	Routine	Range 0-18	NR	NR	NR	NR	NR	NR	NR	NR	NR	NR	NR	NR
Bhuripanyo 1995 7622976	Routine	≥15	NR	A 100% (implied)	NR	NR	NR	NR	NR	NR	NR	NR	NR	NR
Bhuripanyo 1990 2345323	Routine	44 (15-77)	36	A 100% (implied)	NR	NR	NR	NR	NR	NR	NR	NR	NR	NR
Bhuripanyo 1995 7629451	Routine	NR	NR	A 100% (implied)	NR	NR	NR	NR	NR	NR	NR	NR	NR	NR
Bhuripanyo 1992 1293256	Routine	59 (40-77)	67	A 100% (implied)	NR	NR	NR	NR	NR	NR	NR	NR	NR	NR
Bouillot 1996 8891616	Routine	49 (15-99)	56	NR	NR	NR	NR	NR	NR	NR	NR	NR	NR	NR
Burk 1992 1557263	Routine	Range 3-16	NR	NR	NR	NR	NR	NR	NR	NR	NR	NR	NR	NR
Bushick 1989 2585157	Routine	NR	NR	NR	1, 2	NR	NR	NR	NR	NR	NR	NR	NR	NR
Carliner 1986 3719447	Per protocol	59 (40-88)	70	NR	NR	NR	NR	NR	NR	NR	NR	NR	NR	NR
Charpak 1988 3339918	Per protocol	Range <35->75	36	NR	NR	3%	20%	NR	NR	NR	NR	11% "Lung disease"	NR	6% "Kidney disease"

Author Year PMID	Arm	Age, y Mean (Range)	Male, %	Race	ASA	Diabetes	CHD/CAD/CHF	Stroke/TIA	Arrhythmia	HTN	Obesity	COPD	Asthma	CKD
Charpak 1988 3383317	Per protocol	<35->75	36	NR	NR	3%	20%	NR	NR	NR	NR	NR	NR	NR
Correll 2009 19417620	Per protocol	Mean 66	50	NR	NR	17%	11% MI, 6% Angina, 8% CAD, 11% CHF	4%	NR	49%	NR	NR	NR	7%
Gabriel 2000 10960200	Routine	6 ± 3	NR	NR	NR	NR	NR	NR	NR	NR	NR	NR	NR	NR
Gold 1992 1739358	Per protocol	47 (14-88)	30	NR	1-3	NR	NR	NR	NR	NR	NR	NR	NR	NR
Golub 1992 1595835	Routine	46 (17-92)	38	NR	1-3	NR	NR	NR	NR	NR	NR	NR	NR	NR
Haug 1999 9915390	Routine	23 (15-54)	48	NR	NR	NR	NR	NR	NR	NR	NR	NR	NR	NR
Hoare 1993 8289005	Routine	Range 2-15	NR	NR	NR	NR	NR	NR	NR	NR	NR	NR	NR	NR
Ipp 2011 21926874	Routine	15 (12-18)	27	NR	NR	NR	NR	NR	NR	NR	NR	NR	NR	NR
Johnson 1988 3175862	Routine	64 ± 12	42	NR	NR	NR	NR	NR	NR	NR	NR	NR	NR	NR
Johnson 2002 12190758	Routine	57 (32-90)	43	NR	NR	NR	NR	NR	NR	NR	NR	NR	NR	NR
Kahn 2008 18349183	Routine	NR	0	NR	NR	NR	NR	NR	NR	NR	NR	NR	NR	NR
Kaplan 1985 3999339	Routine	NR	NR	NR	NR	NR	NR	NR	NR	NR	NR	NR	NR	NR
Lafferty 2001 11528304	Routine	55 ± 19	34	NR	NR	NR	NR	NR	NR	NR	NR	NR	NR	NR
Lawrence 1988 3377621	Routine	Range 15-19	80	NR	NR	NR	NR	NR	NR	NR	NR	NR	NR	NR

Author Year PMID	Arm	Age, y Mean (Range)	Male, %	Race	ASA	Diabetes	CHD/CAD/CHF	Stroke/TIA	Arrhythmia	HTN	Obesity	COPD	Asthma	CKD
Mallick 2006 17143358	Routine	4 (1 mo-12 y)	62	NR	NR	NR	NR	NR	NR	NR	NR	NR	NR	NR
Malviya 1996 8831334	Routine	15 (10-17)	0	NR	NR	NR	NR	NR	NR	NR	NR	NR	NR	NR
Manning 1987 3679679	Routine	NR	NR	NR	NR	NR	NR	NR	NR	NR	NR	NR	NR	NR
Mantha 2005 15721730	Routine	Median 38 (IQR 32-47)	57	A 100%	NR	NR	NR	NR	NR	NR	NR	NR	NR	NR
Narr 1991 1899710	Routine	NR	NR	NR	1	NR	NR	NR	NR	NR	NR	NR	NR	NR
Nigam 1990 2073764	Routine	Range 3-12	NR	W 63%, B 8%, A 29%	NR	NR	NR	NR	NR	NR	NR	NR	NR	NR
O'Connor 1990 2301750	Routine	Range <1-17	65	NR	NR	NR	NR	NR	NR	NR	NR	NR	NR	NR
Paterson 1983 6867689	Routine	NR	NR	NR	NR	NR	NR	NR	NR	NR	NR	NR	NR	NR
Perez 1995 7718366	Routine	Range 0-98	54	NR	1, 2	NR	NR	NR	NR	NR	NR	NR	NR	NR
Pierre 1998 9704304	Routine	Range 12-21	0	NR	NR	NR	NR	NR	NR	NR	NR	NR	NR	NR
Phillips, 2013 23508220	Routine	<75 (48%)- ≥75 (52%)	48	W 93%, non-W 7%	NR	22%	24%	NR	16%	68%	NR	13% "Chronic lung disease"	NR	NR
Roy 1991 1914052	Routine	Range 1mo-18	63	NR	1, 2	NR	NR	NR	NR	NR	NR	NR	NR	NR
Sane 1977 917629	Routine	0-19	NR	NR	NR	NR	NR	NR	NR	NR	NR	NR	NR	NR
Silvestri 1999 10713868	Per protocol	Mean 54	45	NR	1-5	NR	8% "Cardiac disease"	NR	NR	NR	NR	3% "Respiratory disease"	NR	NR

Author Year PMID	Arm	Age, y Mean (Range)	Male, %	Race	ASA	Diabetes	CHD/CAD/CHF	Stroke/ TIA	Arrhythmia	HTN	Obesity	COPD	Asthma	CKD
Tape 1988 3339483	Routine	67 (24-90)	71	W 95%	NR	29%	35% Prior MI	12% Prior stroke	NR	47%	NR	29%	7%	NR
Van Damme 1997 9158124	Routine	66 ± 10	79	NR	NR	19%	7%, 19% Angina, 7% Unstable angina, 33% Prior MI	NR	NR	31%	NR	NR	NR	NR

Abbreviations: A, Asian; AFib, atrial fibrillation or flutter; ASA, American Surgical Association category; B, black; CABG, coronary artery bypass grafting; CAD, coronary artery disease; CHD, coronary heart disease; CHF, coronary heart failure; CKD, chronic kidney disease; COPD, chronic obstructive pulmonary disease; H, Hispanic; HTN, hypertension; MI, myocardial infarction; NR, not reported; preop, preoperative; TIA, transient ischemic attack; W, white.

C-27

Table C-4. Noncomparative study: Tests by study arm

Author Year PMID	Arm	ECG	CXR	Basic Metabolic	Extended Metabolic	CBC	Hemostasis tests	Urinalysis	Pregnancy Test	Stress Test	Echo	Other
Aghajanian 1991 1923209	Routine						Bleeding time					
Alsumait 2002 12116695	Routine			Na, K, CO2, glucose, BUN, creatinine		Yes	PT-INR, PTT					
Azzam 1996 8712424	Routine								Yes			
Baron 1992 1470961	Routine					Hct						
Bhuripanyo 1995 7622976	Routine					Yes						
Bhuripanyo 1990 2345323	Routine		Yes									
Bhuripanyo 1995 7629451	Routine							Yes				
Bhuripanyo 1992 1293256	Routine	Yes*										
Bouillot 1996 8891616	Routine		Yes									
Burk 1992 1557263	Routine					Yes	PT, PTT, bleeding time					
Bushick 1989 2585157	Routine						PT, aPTT					
Carliner 1986 3719447	Per protocol									Exercise test		

C-28

Author Year PMID	Arm	ECG	CXR	Basic Metabolic	Extended Metabolic	CBC	Hemostasis tests	Urinalysis	Pregnancy Test	Stress Test	Echo	Other
Charpak 1988 3339918	Per protocol	Yes	Yes	Na, K, Cl, HCO3, protein, glucose, creatinine		Hb, platelet	PT, PTT, bleeding time					
Charpak 1988 3383317	Per protocol		Yes									
Correll 2009 19417620	Per protocol	Yes										
Gabriel 2000 10960200	Routine						Bleeding time					
Gold 1992 1739358	Per protocol	Yes										
Golub 1992 1595835	Routine	Ad hoc (73% of patients)	Ad hoc (68% of patients)	SMA-7 (96% of patients)	SMA-12 (Ad hoc 56% of patients): P, Ca, SGOT, GGT, uric acid, total bilirubin, total protein, Alb, LDH, ALP, cholesterol	99% of patients	PT, PTT (89% of patients had each)	99% of patients				
Haug 1999 9915390	Routine	≥40 yo	≥40 yo	Glucose		Yes		Yes	Yes			
Hoare 1993 8289005	Routine					Hb						
Ipp 2011 21926874	Routine	Yes										
Johnson 1988 3175862	Routine	≥40 yo				Yes		Yes				
Johnson 2002 12190758	Routine			Na, K, BUN, creatinine, glucose								

Author Year PMID	Arm	ECG	CXR	Basic Metabolic	Extended Metabolic	CBC	Hemostasis tests	Urinalysis	Pregnancy Test	Stress Test	Echo	Other
Kahn 2008 18349183	Routine								Yes			
Kaplan 1985 3999339	Routine					Yes						
Lafferty 2001 11528304	Routine	Yes	Yes	Na, K, creatinine		Hb, WBC						
Lawrence 1988 3377621	Routine							Yes				
Mallick 2006 17143358	Routine			Electrolytes, BUN		Yes						
Malviya 1996 8831334	Routine								Yes			
Manning 1987 3679679	Routine						PT, PTT					
Mantha 2005 15721730	Routine	Yes	Yes	Na, K, BUN, creatinine, glucose		Hb, WBC						HIV
Narr 1991 1899710	Routine			K, glucose	AST	Hb, platelets						
Nigam 1990 2073764	Routine					Hb						Sickle cell if of Afro-Caribbean descent
O'Connor 1990 2301750	Routine					Hb, Hct, RBC, WBC		Yes				
Paterson 1983 6867689	Routine	Yes										

Author Year PMID	Arm	ECG	CXR	Basic Metabolic	Extended Metabolic	CBC	Hemostasis tests	Urinalysis	Pregnancy Test	Stress Test	Echo	Other
Perez 1995 7718366	Routine			Na, K, BUN, glucose, creatinine	SGOT, SGPT, ALP, "proteinogram", total protein, GGT, "total biochemical"	Yes	PT, PTT					
Pierre 1998 9704304	Routine								Yes			
Phillips, 2013 23508220	Routine	Yes	Yes	Glucose, possibly others		Yes						No complete list of tests reported. Other tests assumed.
Roy 1991 1914052	Routine					Hb						
Sane 1977 917629	Routine		Yes									
Silvestri 1999 10713868	Per protocol		Yes									
Tape 1988 3339483	Routine		Yes									
Van Damme 1997 9158124	Routine									Dobutamine stress echocardiography and sestamibi tomoscintigraphy		

* Performed at the cardiology unit, department of internal medicine by 2 nurses and interpreted by 3 cardiologists or anesthesiologist

Abbreviations: Alb, albumin; ALP, alkaline phosphatase; BUN, blood urea nitrogen; Ca, calcium; CBC, complete blood count; Cl, chloride; CO2, carbon dioxide; CXR, chest x-ray; ECG, electrocardiogram; Echo, echocardiogram; GGT, gamma-glutamyl transpeptidase; Hb, hemoglobin; HCO3, bicarbonate; Hct, hematocrit; K, potassium; LDH, lactate dehydrogenase; Na, sodium; P, phosphorus; preop, preoperative; PT, prothrombin time; PT-INR, prothrombin time and international normalized ratio; (a)PTT, (activated)partial thromboplastin time; RBC, red blood cell count; SGOT, serum glutamic-oxaloacetic transaminase; SGPT, serum glutamic-pyruvic transaminase; SMA(-7, -12), sequential multiple analysis (-7, -12 items); WBC, white blood cell count; yo, years old

Table C-5. Perioperative complications of cataract surgery

Author Year PMID	Study Design	Outcome	Outcome definition	Arm	N Analyzed	Events (%)	RR (95% CI)
Population: Adults							
Test: Panel*							
Cavallini 2004 15506597	RCT **Risk of Bias** Low	Ophthalmic complication	Intraoperative at time 0	With preoperative testing	638	8 (1%)	0.73 (0.29, 1.78)
				Without preoperative testing	638	11 (2%)	
		Ophthalmic complication	Intraoperative at 1 mo	With preoperative testing	638	5 (1%)	0.83 (0.26, 2.72)
				Without preoperative testing	638	6 (1%)	
		Systemic (nonophthalmic) complication	Postoperative at time 0	With preoperative testing	638	4 (1%)	1.00 (0.26, 3.98)
				Without preoperative testing	638	4 (1%)	
		Systemic (nonophthalmic) complication	Postoperative at 1 mo	With preoperative testing	638	0 (0%)	Not calculated
				Without preoperative testing	638	0 (0%)	
Lira 2001 11558245	RCT Low	Perioperative surgical complications	Total adverse events including cardiovascular, cerebrovascular, pulmonary, and psychiatric adverse events	Routine testing	502	48 (10%)	0.98 (0.67, 1.43)
				Ad hoc testing	503	49 (10%)	
		Acute anxiety	Abrupt onset of a fear of death	Routine testing	502	2 (0.4%)	1.00 (0.14, 7.09)
				Ad hoc testing	503	2 (0.4%)	
		Arrhythmia	New or worsening requiring new or change in treatment	Routine testing	502	1 (0.2%)	Not calculated
				Ad hoc testing	503	0 (0%)	
		Bronchospasm	Wheezing or excessive coughing requiring a bronchodilator or theophylline	Routine testing	502	3 (1%)	1.00 (0.20, 4.94)
				Ad hoc testing	503	3 (1%)	

Author Year PMID	Study Design	Outcome	Outcome definition	Arm	N Analyzed	Events (%)	RR (95% CI)
	Risk of Bias						
		Hypertension	Increase to SBP >179 mm Hg or DBP >109 mm Hg, or new or change in treatment required	Routine testing	502	41 (8%)	0.96 (0.63, 1.44)
				Ad hoc testing	503	43 (9%)	
		Myocardial infarction	New or more severe ischemic angina requiring treatment	Routine testing	502	0 (0%)	Not calculated
				Ad hoc testing	503	1 (0.22%)	
		Transient ischemic attack	Abrupt onset of a focal neurologic deficit lasting < 24 hours and resulting from cerebrovascular ischemia	Routine testing	502	1 (0.2%)	Not calculated
				Ad hoc testing	503	0 (0%)	
Nascimento 2004 1525298 (Followup of Lira 2001)		Intraocular lens in the vitreous	Intraocular lens (not defined) migrates into the vitreous cavity	Routine testing	502	2 (0.4%)	Not calculated
				No testing	503	0 (0%)	
		Iridodialysis	Desinsertion of iris root from the ciliary body	Routine testing	502	1 (0.2%)	1.00 (0.06, 15.98)
				No testing	503	1 (0.2%)	
		Ophthalmic complication	Total postoperative complications: Bullous keratopathy, cystoid macular edema, increased intraocular pressure, chronic iriditis, retina detachment, wound leak, vitreous hemorrhage, endophalmitis (<60 days after surgery)	Routine testing	502	49 (10%)	1.14 (0.77, 1.69)
				No testing	503	43 (9%)	
		Posterior capsular rupture (PCR)	Tear or discontinuity of the posterior capsule	Routine testing	502	32 (6%)	0.94 (0.59, 1.50)
				No testing	503	34 (7%)	
		PCR with vitreous loss	Presence of vitreous in the anterior segment through the PCR tear	Routine testing	502	32 (6%)	1.00 (0.62, 1.61)
				No testing	503	32 (6%)	

C-33

Author Year PMID	Study Design	Outcome	Outcome definition	Arm	N Analyzed	Events (%)	RR (95% CI)
	Risk of Bias						
		Retained lens fragment	Lens fragments migrate into the vitreous cavity through PCR or zonular dehiscense	Routine testing	502	1 (0.2%)	Not calculated
				No testing	503	0 (0%)	
		Zonular rupture	Desinsertion of the zonular apparatus from the lens capsule	Routine testing	502	2 (0.4%)	2.00 (0.18, 22.03)
				No testing	503	1 (0.2%)	
Schein 2000 10639542	RCT Medium	Perioperative surgical complications	Total intraoperative and postoperative (up to 1 wk) adverse events	Routine testing	9624	301 (3%)†	1.00 (0.85, 1.17)
				No testing	9626	301 (3%)	
		Arrhythmia	Intraoperative and postoperative up to 1 wk. New or worsening disturbance of heart rhythm requiring new treatment or a change in treatment (bradycardia, atrial fibrillation, ventricular tachycardia, or other; separate data reported for each type)	Routine testing	9624	75 (1%)	1.03 (0.75, 1.42)
				No testing	9626	73 (1%)	
		Atrial fibrillation	Intraoperative and postoperative up to 1 wk	Routine testing	9624	14 (0.1%)	1.56 (0.67, 3.59)
				No testing	9626	9 (0.1%)	
		Bradycardia	Intraoperative and postoperative up to 1 wk	Routine testing	9624	47 (0.5%)	0.90 (0.61, 1.34)
				No testing	9626	52 (0.5%)	
		Congestive heart failure	Intraoperative and postoperative up to 1 wk. New pulmonary edema on a chest radiograph or a diagnosis of congestive heart failure	Routine testing	9624	5 (0.1%)	1.00 (0.29, 3.45)
				No testing	9626	5 (0.1%)	
		Death	Intraoperative and postoperative up to 1 wk	Routine testing	9624	1 (0.01%)	2 (0.2, 22)

Author Year PMID	Study Design	Outcome	Outcome definition	Arm	N Analyzed	Events (%)	RR (95% CI)
	Risk of Bias						
		Diabetic ketoacidosis	Intraoperative and postoperative up to 1 wk. Hyperglycemia with an increase in the anion gap, metabolic acidosis, and serum or urinary ketones	No testing	9626	2 (0.02%)	
				Routine testing	9624	0 (0%)	Not calculated
		Hospitalization	Unplanned hospital admission	No testing	9626	0 (0%)	
				Routine testing	9624	3 (0.03%)	1.67 (0.4, 7)
				No testing	9626	5 (0.05%)	
		Hypoglycemia	Intraoperative and postoperative up to 1 wk. Blood glucose level low enough to require intravenous dextrose	Routine testing	9624	0 (0%)	Not calculated
				No testing	9626	2 (0.02%)	
		Hypokalemia	Intraoperative and postoperative up to 1 wk	Routine testing	9624	0 (0%)	Not calculated
				No testing	9626	2 (0.02%)	
		Hypotension	Intraoperative and postoperative up to 1 wk. Decrease in systolic pressure to <100 mm Hg, with treatment required	Routine testing	9624	14 (0.1%)	0.70 (0.35, 1.39)
				No testing	9626	20 (0.2%)	
		Myocardial infarction	Intraoperative and postoperative up to 1 wk. Evolving changes in the ST-T segment, new Q waves, or both on an electrocardiogram; symptoms of ischemia plus abnormal serum levels of cardiac enzymes; or symptoms of ischemia plus new left bundle-branch block	Routine testing	9624	5 (0.05%)	1.67 (0.40, 6.97)
				No testing	9626	3 (0.03%)	

Author Year PMID	Study Design	Outcome	Outcome definition	Arm	N Analyzed	Events (%)	RR (95% CI)
	Risk of Bias						
		Myocardial ischemia	Intraoperative and postoperative up to 1 wk. New or more severe chest pain diagnosed as ischemia and requiring treatment	Routine testing	9624	10 (0.1%)	1.43 (0.54, 3.75)
				No testing	9626	7 (0.07%)	
		Oxygen desaturation	Intraoperative and postoperative up to 1 wk. Decrease in oxygen saturation to <90%, with supplemental oxygen required	Routine testing	9624	5 (0.05%)	0.71 (0.23, 2.25)
				No testing	9626	7 (0.07%)	
		Pneumonia	Intraoperative and postoperative up to 1 wk	Routine testing	9624	6 (0.06%)	1.20 (0.37, 3.93)
				No testing	9626	5 (0.05%)	
		Respiratory failure	Intraoperative and postoperative up to 1 wk. Need for mechanical ventilation	Routine testing	9624	1 (0.01%)	1.00 (0.06, 15.99)
				No testing	9626	1 (0.01%)	
		Stroke	Intraoperative and postoperative up to 1 wk. Abrupt onset of a focal neurologic deficit lasting >24 hr	Routine testing	9624	4 (0.04%)	2.00 (0.37, 10.92)
				No testing	9626	2 (0.02%)	
		Transient ischemic attack	Intraoperative and postoperative up to 1 wk. Abrupt onset of a focal neurologic deficit lasting <24 hr and resulting from cerebrovascular ischemia	Routine testing	9624	1 (0.01%)	Not calculated
				No testing	9626	0 (0%)	
		Upper respiratory tract infection	Intraoperative and postoperative up to 1 wk	Routine testing	9624	19 (0.2%)	1.27 (0.64, 2.49)
				No testing	9626	15 (0.2%)	
		Ventricular tachycardia	Intraoperative and postoperative up to 1 wk	Routine testing	9624	1 (0.01%)	1.00 (0.06, 15.99)

Author Year PMID	Study Design	Outcome	Outcome definition	Arm	N Analyzed	Events (%)	RR (95% CI)
Risk of Bias							
				No testing	9626	1 (0.01%)	

*See Table 4 for details of the tests given for each arm.

†"We found no benefit of routine preoperative medical testing when the analysis was stratified according to the participating center or the age, sex, or race of the patient. Similarly, there were no significant differences in event rates when the data were stratified according to coexisting illness, ASA risk class, or self-reported health status". Details provided in table 5 of the article† 9455 patients

Abbreviations: CI, confidence interval; DBP, diastolic blood pressure; RCT, randomized controlled study; RR, relative risk; SBP, systolic blood pressure; wk, week

Table C-6. Procedure cancellations

Author Year PMID	Study Design	Outcome definition	Arm	Test§§	N Analyzed	Events (%)	RR (95% CI)
	Risk of Bias						
Population: Adults							
Surgery: Cataract							
Lira 2001 11558245	RCT	All cancellations regardless of cause	Routine testing	Panel	512	10 (2.0%)	1.00 (0.42, 2.38)
	Low		Ad hoc testing		513	10 (2.0%)	
Schein 2000 10639542	RCT	Operations cancelled and not rescheduled	Routine testing	Panel	9775*	151 (1.5%)‡	0.97 (0.78, 1.21)
	Medium		No testing		9782†	156 (1.6%)§	
Surgery: General/Various							
Wyatt 1989 2729769	rNRS	All cancellations regardless of cause	Per protocol testing	Panel	4058	261 (6.4%)	0.93 (0.76, 1.14)
	High		Elective testing		1834	127 (6.9%)	
Wyatt 1989 2729769	rNRS	All cancellations regardless of cause	Per protocol testing	CXR	4058‖	1 (0.02%)¶	Not calculated
	High		Elective testing		1834‖	3 (0.2%)¶	
Wyatt 1989 2729769	rNRS	All cancellations regardless of cause	Per protocol testing	ECG	4058**	5 (0.1%)††	Not calculated
	High		Elective testing		1834**	4 (0.2%)††	
Wyatt 1989 2729769	rNRS	All cancellations regardless of cause	Per protocol testing	"Lab tests"	4058‡‡	38 (0.9%)	Not calculated
	High		Elective testing		1834‡‡	41 (2.2%)	
Population: Pediatrics							
Surgery: General/Various							
Meneghini 1998 9483592	rNRS	Cancellation of surgery due to abnormal test	Routine testing	Panel	1884	0 (0%)	Not calculated
	High		No testing		8772	0 (0%)	

C-38

Author Year PMID	Study Design	Outcome definition	Arm	Test§§	N Analyzed	Events (%)	RR (95% CI)
Risk of Bias							
		Cancellation of surgery regardless of reason	Routine testing	Panel	1884	64 (3.4%)	1.04 (0.80, 1.36)
			No testing		8772	287 (3.3%)	

*9456 patients
† 9455 patients
‡ 145 patients (some of whom had operation in other eye not cancelled)
§ 153 patients (some of whom had operation in other eye not cancelled)
|| Total in group, not total who had a CXR
¶ 3 of 4 cancellations (total) had a positive pulmonary history
** Total in group, not total who had an ECG
†† All had a positive history of cardiac disease
‡‡ Total in group, not total who had a lab test
§§ See Table 4 for details of the tests given for each arm.
Abbreviations: CI, confidence interval; CXR, chest x-ray; ECG, electrocardiogram; RCT, randomized controlled study; rNRS, retrospective nonrandomized (comparative) study; RR, relative risk

Table C-7. Perioperative complications of general or various surgeries

Author Year PMID	Study Design	Outcome	Outcome definition	Arm	N Analyzed	Events (%)	RR (95% CI)
	Risk of Bias						
Population: Adults							
Test: Panel*							
Almanaseer 2005 15528897	rNRS	Angina	Not further defined	Per protocol testing	314	1 (0.3%)	0.83 (0.05, 13.23)
	High			Elective testing	261	1 (0.4%)	
		Cardiac death	Not further defined	Per protocol testing	314	1 (0.3%)	0.83 (0.05, 13.23)
				Elective testing	261	1 (0.4%)	
		Congestive heart failure	Not further defined	Per protocol testing	314	4 (1.3%)	0.42 (0.13, 1.36)
				Elective testing	261	8 (3.1%)	
		Death	Cardiac plus noncardiac death	Per protocol testing	314	1 (0.3%)	0.28 (0.03, 2.65)
				Elective testing	261	3 (1.1%)	
		Myocardial infarction	Not further defined	Per protocol testing	314	1 (0.3%)	Not calculated
				Elective testing	261	0 (0%)	
		Pneumonia	Not further defined	Per protocol testing	314	2 (0.6%)	0.21, 0.04, 0.97)
				Elective testing	261	8 (3.1%)	
		Renal failure	Not further defined	Per protocol testing	314	4 (1.3%)	1.11 (0.25, 4.91)
				Elective testing	261	3 (1.1%)	
		Respiratory failure	Not further defined	Per protocol testing	314	5 (1.6%)	0.59 (0.19, 1.85)
				Elective testing	261	7 (2.7%)	
		Stroke	Not further defined	Per protocol testing	314	2 (0.6%)	Not calculated
				Elective testing	261	0 (0%)	
Falcone 2003 14689407	RCT	Dobutamine stress	Cardiovascular complications	Routine	46	1 (2%)	0.38 (0.04, 3.57)
	Low			No testing	53	3 (6%)	
		ECG	Cardiac Death	Routine	46	0 (0%)	Not calculated
				No testing	53	0 (0%)	
			Death	Routine	46	0 (0%)	Not calculated
				No testing	53	1 (2%)	
Finegan 2005 15983141	pNRS	Perioperative surgical complications	Nonspecified	Routine testing	507	4 (0.8%)	0.43 (0.13, 1.40)
	High			Ad hoc testing	431	8 (1.9%)	
		Death	Not further defined	Routine testing	507	0 (0%)	Not calculated
				Ad hoc testing	431	4 (0.9%)	

C-40

Author Year PMID	Study Design	Outcome	Outcome definition	Arm	N Analyzed	Events (%)	RR (95% CI)
	Risk of Bias						
		Renal failure	Not further defined	Routine testing	507	0 (0%)	Not calculated
				Ad hoc testing	431	4 (0.9%)	
Larocque 1994 7922901	rNRS High	Perioperative surgical complications	Total "morbidities" including infectious, cardiac, respiratory, surgical trauma, surgical bleeding, surgical increased intraocular pressure, gastrointestinal	Per protocol testing	501	46 (9.2%)	0.71 (0.49, 1.01)
				Ad hoc testing	492	64 (13%)	
		Angina	Not further defined	Per protocol testing	501	3 (0.6%)	0.98 (0.20, 4.84)
				Ad hoc testing	492	3 (0.6%)	
		Arrhythmia	Not further defined	Per protocol testing	501	2 (0.4%)	0.65 (0.11, 3.90)
				Ad hoc testing	492	3 (0.6%)	
		Bleeding	Not further defined	Per protocol testing	501	3 (0.6%)	0.74 (0.17, 3.27)
				Ad hoc testing	492	4 (0.8%)	
		Conduction block	Not further defined	Per protocol testing	501	1 (0.2%)	Not calculated
				Ad hoc testing	492	0 (0%)	
		Congestive heart failure	Not further defined	Per protocol testing	501	2 (0.4%)	0.65 (0.11, 3.90)
				Ad hoc testing	492	3 (0.6%)	
		Death	Not further defined	Per protocol testing	501	0 (0%)	Not calculated
				Ad hoc testing	492	2 (0.4%)	
		Death, attributable to test	Attributable to preoperative laboratory investigation(s), either done or not done	Per protocol testing	501	0 (0%)	Not calculated
				Ad hoc testing	492	0 (0%)	
		Fever	Implementation of guidelines for preoperative laboratory investigations in patients scheduled to undergo elective surgery	Per protocol testing	501	8 (1.6%)	1.31 (0.46, 3.75)
				Ad hoc testing	492	6 (1.2%)	
		Gastrointestinal bleed	Not further defined	Per protocol testing	501	0 (0%)	Not calculated
				Ad hoc testing	492	1 (0.2%)	
		Increased intraocular pressure	Not further defined	Per protocol testing	501	4 (0.8%)	0.65 (0.19, 2.31)
				Ad hoc testing	492	6 (1.2%)	

Author Year PMID	Study Design	Outcome	Outcome definition	Arm	N Analyzed	Events (%)	RR (95% CI)
	Risk of Bias						
		Morbidity attributable to test	Attributable to preoperative laboratory investigation(s), either done or not done	Per protocol testing	501	0 (0%)	Not calculated
				Ad hoc testing	492	0 (0%)	
		Pneumonia	Not further defined	Per protocol testing	501	0 (0%)	Not calculated
				Ad hoc testing	492	7 (1.4%)	
		Seizure	Not further defined	Per protocol testing	501	1 (0.2%)	0.98 (0.06, 15.7)
				Ad hoc testing	492	1 (0.2%)	
		Sepsis	Not further defined	Per protocol testing	501	1 (0.2%)	0.98 (0.06, 15.7)
				Ad hoc testing	492	1 (0.2%)	
		Shortness of breath	Not further defined	Per protocol testing	501	0 (0%)	Not calculated
				Ad hoc testing	492	5 (1.0%)	
		Stroke	Not further defined	Per protocol testing	501	1 (0.2%)	0.98 (0.06, 15.66)
				Ad hoc testing	492	1 (0.2%)	
		Urinary tract infection	Not further defined	Per protocol testing	501	5 (1.0%)	1.23 (0.33, 4.54)
				Ad hoc testing	492	4 (0.8%)	
Mignonsin, 1996 8762245	p,rNRS High	Bleeding	Hemorrhage (900-1700 mL) due to defective hemostasis	Routine	200	1 (1%)	Not calculated
				Per protocol	200	0 (0%)	
		Delayed awakening	30 minutes	Routine	200	0 (0%)	Not calculated
				Per protocol	200	1 (0.5%)	
		Death	Not further defined	Routine	200	0 (0%)	Not calculated
				Per protocol	200	0 (0%)	
		Postoperative morbidity	Complication inducing sequelae (or death)	Routine	200	0 (0%)	Not calculated
				Per protocol	200	0 (0%)	
Population: Pediatrics							
Meneghini 1998 9483592	rNRS High	Perioperative surgical complications	Minor	Routine testing	1884	292 (15%)	1.21 (1.08, 1.36)
				No testing	8772	1123 (13%)	
			Major	Routine testing	1884	2 (0.1%)	2.33 (0.43, 12.7)
				No testing	8772	4 (0.05%)	
		Fever	As a minor complication	Routine testing	1884	8 (0.4%)	0.91 (0.43, 1.93)
				No testing	8772	41 (0.5%)	
		Laryngospasm	As a minor complication	Routine testing	1884	24 (1.3%)	1.77 (1.11, 2.83)

C-42

Author Year PMID	Study Design	Outcome	Outcome definition	Arm	N Analyzed	Events (%)	RR (95% CI)
	Risk of Bias						
		Mild perioperative oxygen desaturation	As a minor complication	No testing	8772	63 (0.7%)	
				Routine testing	1884	196 (10%)	1.07 (0.92, 1.24)
				No testing	8772	854 (10%)	
		Persistent vomiting	As a minor complication	Routine testing	1884	39 (2.1%)	1.76 (1.22, 2.54)
				No testing	8772	103 (1.2%)	
		Restlessness	As a minor complication	Routine testing	1884	21 (1.1%)	3.91 (2.19, 6.97)
				No testing	8772	25 (0.3%)	
		Wound complications	As a minor complication	Routine testing	1884	4 (0.2%)	0.51 (0.18, 1.44)
				No testing	8772	37 (0.4%)	

* See Table 4 for details of the tests given for each arm.

Abbreviations: CI, confidence interval; NR, not reported; pNRS, prospective nonrandomized (comparative) study; p,rNRS, combined pro- and retrospective nonrandomized (comparative) study; RCT, randomized controlled study; rNRS, retrospective nonrandomized (comparative) study; RR, relative risk

Table C-8. Return to the operating room

Author Year PMID	Study Design	Outcome definition	Arm	Test*	N Analyzed	Events (%)	RR (95% CI)
		Risk of Bias					
Surgery: **General/Various**							
Population: Adults							
Larocque 1994 7922901	rNRS	Return to the operating room (not further defined)	Per protocol testing	Panel	501	1 (0.2%)	0.25 (0.03, 2.19)
	High		Ad hoc testing		492	4 (0.8%)	

* See Table 4 for details of the tests given for each arm.

Abbreviations: CI, confidence interval; rNRS, retrospective nonrandomized (comparative) study; RR, relative risk

Table C-9. Unplanned hospital admission

Author Year PMID	Study Design	Outcome definition	Arm	Test*	N Analyzed	Events (%)	RR (95% CI)
	Risk of Bias						
Surgery: General/Various							
Population: Adults							
Chung 2009 19151274	RCT	Hospital revisit in ≤7 days	Per protocol testing	Panel	527	27 (5%)	0.4 (0.2, 0.9)
	Low		No testing		499	11 (2%)	
Surgery: Orthopedic							
Population: Adults							
Mancuso 1999 10203622	rNRS	Hospital admission	Routine testing	Panel	361	10 (3%)	0.86 (0.35, 2.08)
	High		Per protocol testing		279	9 (3%)	

* See Table 4 for details of the tests given for each arm.

Abbreviations: CI, confidence interval; rNRS, retrospective nonrandomized (comparative) study; RR, relative risk

Table C-10. Prolonged hospital admission

Author Year PMID	Study Design	Outcome definition	Arm	Test*	N Analyzed	Events (%)	RR (95% CI)
	Risk of Bias						
Surgery: General/Various							
Population: Adults							
Larocque 1994 7922901	rNRS	Prolonged hospital admission (not further defined)	Per protocol testing	Panel	501	1 (0.2%)	Not calculated
	High						
			Ad hoc testing		492	4 (1%)	
Population: Pediatrics							
Meneghini 1998 9483592	rNRS	Longer hospital stay than expected	Routine testing	Panel	1884	51 (2.7%)	0.89 (0.66, 1.20)
	High						
			No testing		8772	266 (3.0%)	

* See Table 4 for details of the tests given for each arm.

Abbreviations: CI, confidence interval; rNRS, retrospective nonrandomized (comparative) study; RR, relative risk

Table C-11. Length of hospital stay (continuous outcome)

Author Year PMID	Study Design	Outcome definition	Arm	Test*	N Analyzed	Mean (Range)	P-value
Risk of Bias							
Surgery: General/Various							
Population: Adults							
Almanaseer 2005 15528897	rNRS	Length of hospital stay in days	Per protocol testing	Panel	314	5.6 (1, 30)	0.055
	High		Elective testing		261	6.5 (1, 42)	
Population: Pediatrics							
Leonard 1975 1095116	RCT	Length of hospital stay in days	Routine Hb and metabolic panel	Panel	386	3.7 (NR)	>0.1
	Medium		Routine Hb only		403	3.4 (NR)	

* See Table 4 for details of the tests given for each arm.

Abbreviations: NR, not reported; rNRS, retrospective (nonrandomized) comparative study

Table C-12. Procedure or anesthesia delay

Author Year PMID	Study Design	Outcome definition	Arm	Test*	N Analyzed	Events (%)	RR (95% CI)
		Risk of Bias					
Population: Adults							
Surgery: **General/Various**							
Almanaseer 2005 15528897	rNRS	Procedure or anesthesia delay (not further defined)	Per protocol testing	Panel	314	16 (5.1%)	1.33 (0.61, 2.88)
	High		Elective testing		261	10 (3.8%)	
			Per protocol testing		279	1%	

* See Table 4 for details of the tests given for each arm.

Abbreviations: CI, confidence interval; rNRS, retrospective nonrandomized (comparative) study; RR, relative risk

C-48

Table C-13. Perioperative complications of vascular surgeries

Author Year PMID	Study Design	Outcome	Outcome definition	Arm	N Analyzed	Events (%)	RR (95% CI)
	Risk of Bias						
Population: Adults							
Test: Panel*							
Falcone 2003 14689407	RCT	Dobutamine stress	Cardiovascular complications	Routine	46	1 (2%)	0.38 (0.04, 3.57)
	Low			No testing	53	3 (6%)	
		ECG	Cardiac Death	Routine	46	0 (0%)	Not calculated
				No testing	53	0 (0%)	
			Death	Routine	46	0 (0%)	Not calculated
				No testing	53	1 (2%)	

* See Table 4 for details of the tests given for each arm.

Abbreviations: CI, confidence interval; RCT, randomized controlled study; RR, relative risk

Table C-14. Perioperative complications of tonsillectomy

Author Year PMID	Study Design	Outcome	Outcome definition	Arm	N Analyzed	Events (%)	RR (95% CI)
Risk of Bias							
Population: Pediatrics							
Test: Panel*							
Zwack 1997 9051441	rNRS	Bleeding	Peri/postoperative bleeding (<24 hr or >24 hr postoperative)	Routine testing	1750	22 (1.3%)†	2.06 (1.09, 3.91)
	High			Per protocol testing	2624	16 (0.7%)‡	

* See Table 4 for details of the tests given for each arm.

† 21/22 had normal laboratory tests; one had a minimally abnormal PT (0.1 second above normal).

‡ 8 had no preoperative PT/PTT. The other 8 had normal PT/PTT (screened for suspicious history

Abbreviations: CI, confidence interval; hr, hour; rNRS, retrospective nonrandomized (comparative) study; RR, relative risk

Table C-15. Change in surgical technique

Population	Procedure	Test Category	Tests	No. Studies (RoB)	No. Patients	Range of %, Across Studies	Combined % (95% CI), by Test Category
Adult	Various/general	Hemostasis tests		1 (1 M)	3089	0%	0.0% (0.0%, 0.3%)
		Combined panel	Various*	2 (1L, 1M)	6650	0-0.03%	0.0% (0.0%, 0.1%)
	Vascular	Stress test	Dobutamine stress echocardiography and sestamibi tomoscintigraphy	1 (1 M)	150	0.7%	0.7% (0.1%, 4.8%)
Pediatric	Various/general	CXR		1 (1 L)	1500	0%	0.0% (0.0%, 0.5%)

* ECG, CXR, basic metabolic and CBC, hemostasis; Biochemical panel (not further described)

Abbreviations: CXR, chest x-ray; L, low risk of bias; M, medium risk of bias; RoB, the number of studies at each risk of bias level

Table C-16. Change in anesthetic management

Population	Procedure	Test Category	Tests	No. Studies (RoB)	No. Patients	Range of % Across Studies	Combined % (95% CI), by Test Category
Adult	Various/general	Metabolic panel	Basic and extended panel	1 (1M)	2784	0.2%	3.3% (2.9%, 3.9%)
			Electrolytes	1 (1L)	1001	10%	
			Creatinine	1 (1L)	995	5.5%	
			Glucose	1 (1L)	705	2.1%	
		CXR		4 (3L, 1M)	12,104	0.5-3.7%	2.3% (2.0%, 2.6%)
		ECG		1 (1L)	1610	7.3%	7.3% (6.5%, 9.5%)
		CBC	Hb	1 (1L)	2138	6.5%	6.0% (5.4%-7.5%)
			Platelets	1 (1L)	290	1.7%	
		Hemostasis tests	PT or PTT ± CBC	2 (1L, 1M)	4976	0-2.9%	1.1% (0.9%, 1.5%)
			Bleeding time	1 (1L)	21	4.8%	
		Combined panel	Various*	5 (4L, 1H)	4640	0% (4 studies); 9.0% (1 study)	7.5% (7.2%, 9.0%)
Pediatric	Various/general	CXR		1 (1L)	1500	2.3%	2.3% (1.7%, 3.3%)
		CBC	Hb or Hct	2 (2L)	2238	0%	0.0% (0.0%, 0.4%)
		Combined panel	Basic metabolic and CBC	1 (1L)	342	0%	0.0% (0.0%, 2.3%)
		Pregnancy test		2 (2L)	651	0-1.0%	0.3% (0.1%, 1.2%)

* Basic metabolic and CBC; basic metabolic, and extended metabolic, CBC, hemostasis tests, urinalysis (and ad hoc ECG and CXR); ECG, CBC, and urinalysis; ECG, CBC, basic metabolic, CBC, hemostasis tests.

Abbreviations: CBC, complete blood count; CXR, chest x-ray; ECG, electrocardiogram H, high risk of bias; Hb, hemoglobin; Hct, hematocrit; L, low risk of bias; M, medium risk of bias; PT, prothrombin time; PTT, partial thromboplastin time; RoB, the number of studies at each risk of bias level

Table C-17. Procedure cancellations

Population	Procedure	Test Category	Tests	No. Studies (RoB)	No. Patients	Range of %, Across Studies	Combined % (95% CI), by Test Category
Adult	ECT	CBC		1 (1 H)	73	0%	0.0% (0.0%, 11.2%)
		CXR		1 (1 H)	64	0%	0.0% (0.0%, 12.8%)
		ECG		1 (1 H)	73	1.4%	1.4% (0.2%, 10.0%)
		Metabolic panel	Electrolytes and creatinine	1 (1 H)	73	0%	0.0% (0.0%, 11.2%)
		Combined panel	All test above	1 (1 H)	73	1.4%	1.4% (0.2%, 10.0%)
	Various/general	Stress test	Exercise test	1 (1 L)	100	4.0%	4.0% (1.5%, 11.3%)
		CXR		2 (1 M, 1 H)	5159	0.02-0.3%	0.1% (0.0%, 0.2%)
		ECG		4 (2 L, 2 H)	5149	0.12-1.5%	0.2% (0.1%, 0.4%)
		Combined panel	Various*	8 (4 L, 1 M, 3 H)	13,090	0-6.4%	2.1% (1.9%, 2.5%)
		Hemostasis tests	PT/INR	1 (1 L)	1546	0%	0.0% (0.0%, 0.5%)
		Urinalysis		1 (1 M)	917	0%	0.0% (0.0%, 0.9%)
		Pregnancy test		1 (1 L)	2593	0%	0.0% (0.0%, 0.3%)
		"Lab tests"		1 (1 H)	4058	0.94%	0.9% (0.7%, 1.3%)
	Head & Neck/ENT	Combined panel	ECG, CXR, basic metabolic, CBC, urinalysis, pregnancy test	1 (1 L)	380	0%	0.0% (0.0%, 2.1%)
	Neurosurgery	Combined panel	EGC, CXR, basic metabolic, CBC, HIV	1 (1 H)	127	0%	0.0% (0.0%, 6.4%)
	Orthopedic	Hemostasis tests	PT and PTT	1 (1 M)	640	0%	0.0% (0.0%, 1.3%)
	Vascular	Stress test	Dobutamine stress echocardiography and sestamibi tomoscintigraphy	1 (1 M)	150	2.0%	2.0% (0.7%, 6.4%)
	Cataract	Combined panel	Various‡	2 (1 L, 1 M)	9958	1.5-2.0%	1.6% (1.4%, 1.9%)
Pediatric	Various/general	CBC	Hct	1 (1 L)	238	0%	0.0% (0.0%, 3.4%)
		Combined panel	Various†	3 (2 L, 1 H))	2712	0%	0.0% (0.0%, 0.3%)
		Pregnancy test		2 (2 L)	1008	0.5%	0.5% (0.2%, 1.2%)
	Head & Neck/ENT	CBC	Hb	1 (1 L)	372	0.5%	0.5% (0.1%, 2.2%)
	Tonsillectomy	Hemostasis tests	Bleeding time	2 (2 L)	2473	0-0.1%	0.04% (0.01%, 0.3%)

Population	Procedure	Test Category	Tests	No. Studies (RoB)	No. Patients	Range of %, Across Studies	Combined % (95% CI), by Test Category
		CBC	Hb	1 (1 L)	250	0%	0.0% (0.0%, 3.2%)
		Combined panel	CBC and hemostasis	1 (1 L)	1603	0.06%	0.1% (0.01%, 0.4%)
		Sickle cell		1 (1 L)	21	0%	0.0% (0.1%, 41.0%)

* ECG, CBC, urinalysis; basic metabolic, and extended metabolic, CBC, hemostasis tests, urinalysis (and ad hoc ECG and CXR); CBC, rapid plasma regain; basic metabolic, CBC; basic metabolic, CBC, hemostasis tests; basic metabolic, extended metabolic, CBC; ECG, CXR, basic metabolic, CBC, hemostasis tests; CBC, urinalysis, creatine phosphokinase test, cholinesterase; ECG, CXR, basic metabolic, extended metabolic, CBC, hemostasis, urinalysis

‡ EGC, basic metabolic, CBC; ECG, basic metabolic, CBC, urinalysis

†CBC, urinalysis; basic metabolic, CBC; CBC, urinalysis, CPK, cholinesterase

Abbreviations: CBC, complete blood count; CXR, chest x-ray; ECG, electrocardiogram; ECT, electroconvulsive therapy; ENT, ear, nose and throat; H, high risk of bias; Hb, hemoglobin; Hct, hematocrit; HIV, human immunodeficiency virus; L, low risk of bias; M, medium risk of bias; PT, prothrombin time; PTT, partial thromboplastin time; RoB, the number of studies at each risk of bias level.

Table C-18. Procedure or anesthetic delay

Population	Procedure	Test Category	Tests	No. Studies (RoB)	No. Patients	Range of %, Across Studies	Combined % (95% CI), by Test Category
Adult	Cataract	Combined panel	Various [complete list not reported]	1 (1 L)	530	3.6%	3.6% (2.4%, 5.9%)
	Various/general	"Biochemical panel"		1 (1 M)	2784	0.2%	0.2% (0.1%, 0.4%)
		Stress test	Exercise test	2 (2 L)	300	1.0-11%	4.3% (2.6%, 7.9%)
		CXR		1 (1 L)	933	2.0%	2.0% (1.3%, 3.3%)
		ECG		1 (1 L)	284	1.1%	1.1% (0.3%, 3.3%)
		Combined panel	Various*	6 (2 L, 1 M, 3 H)	5268	0-5.1%	0.4% (0.3%, 0.6%)
		Hemostasis tests	PT or PTT ± CBC	2 (1 L, 1 M)	4635	0-0.1%	0.1% (0.0%, 0.2%)
		Pregnancy test		1 (1 L)	2593	0.2%	0.2% (0.1%, 0.5%)
	Head & Neck/ENT	Combined panel	ECG, CXR, basic metabolic, CBC, urinalysis, pregnancy test	1 (1 L)	380	0.5%	0.5% (0.1%, 2.1%)
	Neurosurgery	Combined panel	EGC, CXR, basic metabolic, CBC, HIV	1 (1 H)	127	0%	0.0% (0.0%, 6.4%)
	Orthopedic	Hemostasis tests	PT and PTT	1 (1 M)	640	0.2%	0.2% (0.0%, 1.1%)
		Urinalysis		1 (1 L)	200	0.5%	0.5% (0.1%, 3.6%)
		Combined panel	Various*	1 (1 M)	640	1.6%	1.6% (0.8%, 3.0%)
	Vascular	Stress test	Dobutamine stress echocardiography and sestamibi tomoscintigraphy	1 (1 M)	150	3.3%	
		CXR		1 (1 M)	341	1.2%	
Pediatric	Various/general	CXR		1 (1 L)	1500	0.7%	0.7% (0.4%, 1.3%)
		CBC	Hb ±MCV, WBC	2 (2 L)	2484	0-0.4%	0.2% (0.1%, 0.5%)
		Pregnancy test		2 (2 L)	651	0-2.3%	1.5% (0.8%, 2.9%)
		Urinalysis		1 (1 L)	453	0.4%	0.4% (0.1%, 1.8%)
	Head & Neck/ENT	CBC	Hb	1 (1 L)	372	2.7%	2.7% (1.5%, 5.2%)
	Orthopedic	Combined panel	ECG, Echocardiogram	1 (1 L)	212	0.9%	0.9% (0.2%, 3.8%)

* ECG, CBC, urinalysis; basic metabolic, and extended metabolic, CBC, hemostasis tests, urinalysis (and ad hoc ECG and CXR); CBC, rapid plasma reagin; basic metabolic, CBC; basic metabolic, CBC, hemostasis tests; basic metabolic, extended metabolic, CBC; ECG, stress test, echocardiogram, cardiac workup, coronary angiography

Abbreviations: CBC, complete blood count; CXR, chest x-ray; ECG, electrocardiogram; ENT, ear, nose and throat; H, high risk of bias; Hb, hemoglobin; L, low risk of bias; M, medium risk of bias; MCV, mean corpuscular volume; PT, prothrombin time; PTT, partial thromboplastin time; RoB, the number of studies at each risk of bias level; WBC, white blood count

Table C-19. Noncomparative studies: Change in anesthetic management

Author, Year, PMID	Study Design	Outcome Definition	Arm	N Analyzed	Counts (%)
Population: Adults					
Surgery:					
General/Various					
Test: Metabolic Panel					
Perez 1995 7718366	Retrospective cohort	Change in anesthetic technique	Routine	2784	5 (0.2%)
Charpak 1988 3339918	Prospective cohort	Treatment was instituted or anesthetic management influenced	Per Protocol (Test: Electrolytes)	1001	105 (10%)
			Per Protocol (Test: Creatinine)	995	55 (5.5%)
			Per Protocol (Test: Glucose)	705	15 (2.1%)
Test: CXR					
Charpak 1988 3383317	Prospective cohort	"Anesthetic management was influenced"; CXR considered useful per anesthesiologist	Per Protocol	1101	27 (2.5%)
Silvestri 1999 10713868	Prospective cohort	Change from general or regional anesthesia	Per Protocol	6111	226 (3.7%)
Bouillot 1996 8891616	Prospective cohort	Changes in surgical "policy" or anesthesia	Routine	3959	13[2] (~0.5%)
Bhuripanyo 1990 2345323	Retrospective cohort	NR	Routine	933	7 (0.8%)[3]
Test: ECG					
Charpak 1988 3339918	Prospective cohort	Treatment was instituted or anesthetic management influenced	Per Protocol	1610	117 (7.3%)
Test: CBC					
Charpak 1988 3339918	Prospective cohort	Treatment was instituted or anesthetic management influenced	Per Protocol (Test: Hb)	2138	140 (6.5%)
			Per Protocol (Test: Platelets)	290	5 (1.7%)
Test: Hemostasis Tests					
Charpak 1988 3339918	Prospective cohort	Treatment was instituted or anesthetic management influenced	Per Protocol (Test: PT)	935	27 (2.9%)
			Per Protocol (Test: PTT)	952	27 (2.8%)
			Per Protocol (Test: Bleeding)	21	1 (4.8%)
Perez 1995 7718366	Retrospective cohort	Change in anesthetic technique	Routine (Test: PT, PTT, CBC)	3089	0 (0%)

[2] In Table IV Total = "3", but 2+2+6+3=13 and 13/3959 ~ 0.5%
[3] Subgroup analysis shows a significant difference between <45 and ≥4, P<0.0001

C-56

Author, Year, PMID	Study Design	Outcome Definition	Arm	N Analyzed	Counts (%)
Test: Panel					
Johnson 2002 12190758	Prospective cohort	Implied	Routine	100	0 (0%)
Golub 1992 1595835	Retrospective cohort	NR	Routine	325	0 (0%)
Johnson 1988 3175862	Prospective cohort	Original plan for anesthesia was changed. "The usual change involved adding intravenous sedation to local anesthesia, which required an anesthesiologist."	Routine	212	0 (0%)
Alsumait 2002 12116695	Prospective cohort	"Change in the management… by the anesthetist"	Routine	137	0 (0%)
Charpak 1988 3339918	Prospective cohort	Treatment was instituted or anesthetic management influenced	Per Protocol	3866	347 (9.0%)
Population: Pediatrics					
Test: CXR					
Sane 1977 917629	Prospective cohort	Use of cardiac monitors, increased observation time, assisted respiration, respiratory tract suction.	Routine	1500	34 (2.3%)
Test: CBC					
Roy 1991 1914052	Retrospective cohort	NR	Routine (Test: Hb)	2000	0 (0%)
Baron 1992 1470961	Retrospective cohort	NR	Routine (Test: Hct)	238	0 (0%)
Test: Panel					
Mallick 2006 17143358	Retrospective cohort	NR	Routine	342	0 (0%)
Test: Pregnancy Test					
Azzam 1996 8712424	Retrospective cohort	1 excluded nitrous oxide (implied), 1 had local anesthesia without sedation	Routine	207	2 (1.0%)
Malviya 1996 8831334	Prospective cohort	Anesthetic or surgical management	Routine	444	0 (0%)

Abbreviations: CBC, complete blood count; CXR, chest x-ray; ECG, electrocardiogram; Hb, hemoglobin; Hct, hematocrit; NR, not reported; PT, prothrombin time; PTT, partial thromboplastin time

Table C-20. Noncomparative studies: Procedure cancellations

Author, Year, PMID	Study Design	Outcome Definition	Arm	N Analyzed	Counts (%)
Population: Adults					
Surgery: ECT					
Test: CBC					
Lafferty 2001 11528304	Cohort (unclear)	NR	Routine	73	0 (0%)
Test: CXR					
Lafferty 2001 11528304	Cohort (unclear)	NR	Routine	62-64	0 (0%)
Test: ECG					
Lafferty 2001 11528304	Cohort (unclear)	NR	Routine	73	1 (1.4%)
Test: Metabolic Panel					
Lafferty 2001 11528304	Cohort (unclear)	NR	Routine	73	0 (0%)
Test: Panel					
Lafferty 2001 11528304	Cohort (unclear)	NR	Routine	73	1 (1.4%)[4]
Surgery: General/Various					
Test: Cardiac Stress Test					
Test: CXR					
Charpak 1987 3383317	Prospective cohort	NR	Per Protocol	1101	3 (0.3%)
Test: ECG					
Correll 2009 19417620	Retrospective cohort	Patients had their case cancelled, and the results of the workup are not known.	Per Protocol	284	2 (0.7%)
Gold 1992 1739358	Retrospective cohort	Surgery postponed because of a preoperative ECG abnormality (right bundle-branch block). Ultimately, the patient did not have surgery despite subsequent evaluation that did not reveal cardiac disease.	Per Protocol	540	1 (0.2%)
Paterson 1983 6867689	Prospective cohort	Operation was canceled	Routine	267	4 (1.5%)[5]
Test: Panel					
Johnson 1988 3175862	Prospective cohort	NR	Routine	212	
Golub 1992 1595835	Retrospective cohort	NR	Routine	325	0 (0%)

[4] ECG revealed AFib which led to AAA repair; judged to no longer need ECT after vascular surgery.
[5] 3/4 had positive responses to questionnaire about cardiovascular symptoms and history. All were >50 years old

C-58

Author, Year, PMID	Study Design	Outcome Definition	Arm	N Analyzed	Counts (%)
Kaplan 1985 3999339	Retrospective cohort	Implied by "alterations in patient care"	Routine	610	0 (0%)
Johnson 2002 12190758	Prospective cohort	Implied	Routine	100	0 (0%)
Alsumait 2002 12116695	Prospective cohort	Implied by "change in the management by surgeon or anesthetist"	Routine	137	0 (0%)
Narr 1991 1899710	Retrospective cohort	Implied	Routine	3782	0 (0%)
Charpak 1988 3339918	Prospective cohort	Surgery was delayed or cancelled	Per Protocol	3866	19 (0.5%)
Test: Hemostasis Tests					
Aghajanian 1991 193209	Retrospective cohort	NR	Routine (Test: PT)	1546	0 (0%)
Test: Urinalysis					
Bhuripanyo 1995 7629451	Prospective cohort	NR	Routine	917	0 (0%)
Test: Pregnancy Test					
Kahn 2008 18349183	Retrospective cohort	NR	Routine	2593	0 (0%)
Surgery: Head & Neck/ ENT					
Test: Panel					
Haug 1999 9915390	Prospective cohort	NR	Routine	380	0 (0%)
Surgery: Neurosurgery					
Test: Panel					
Mantha 2005 15721730	Prospective cohort	Implied	Routine	127[6]	0 (0%)
Surgery: Orthopedic					
Test: Hemostasis Tests					
Bushick 1989 2585157	Retrospective cohort	Implied	Routine	640	0 (0%)
Surgery: Vascular					
Test: Cardiac Stress Test					
Van Damme 1997 9158124	Prospective cohort	Planned repair was cancelled	Routine	150	3 (2.0%)
Population: Pediatrics					
Surgery: General/Various					
Test: CBC					
Baron 1992 1470961	Retrospective cohort	NR	Routine (Test: Hct)	238	0 (0%)
Test: Panel					

[6] Of 1395 tests performed, 37% were indicated

C-59

Author, Year, PMID	Study Design	Outcome Definition	Arm	N Analyzed	Counts (%)[7]
O'Connor 1990 2301750	Retrospective cohort	Surgery cancelled	Routine	486	0 (0%)
Mallick 206 17143358	Retrospective cohort	NR	Routine	342	0 (0%)
Test: Pregnancy Test					
Pierre 1998 9704304	Retrospective cohort	Surgery procedure was postponed	Routine	801	4 (0.5%)[8]
Azzam 1996 8712424	Retrospective cohort	NR	Routine	207	1 (0.5%)
Surgery: Head & Neck/ ENT					
Test: CBC					
Hoare 1993 8289005	Cohort (unclear)	Procedure delay and subsequent failure to have surgery: 1 "failed to attend"; 1 had "further cancellation [due to] gastrointestinal upset"	Routine (Test: Hb)	372	2 (0.5%)
Surgery: Tonsillectomy					
Test: Hemostasis Tests					
Gabriel 2000 10960200	Prospective cohort	NR	Routine	1479	0 (0%)
Manning 1987 3679679	Retrospective cohort	Surgery cancelled due to abnormal PT/PTT	Routine	994	1 (0.1%)
Test: CBC					
Nigam 1990 2073761	Prospective cohort	Due to testing	Routine (Test: Hb)	250	0 (0%)
Test: Panel					
Burk 1992 1557263	Prospective cohort	Patients who did not undergo surgery	Routine	1603	1 (0.06%)
Test: Sickle Cell					
Nigam 1990 2073761	Prospective cohort	Due to testing	Routine	21	0 (0%)

Abbreviations: AAA, abdominal aortic aneurysm; AFib, atrial fibrillation; CABG, coronary artery bypass grafting; CBC, complete blood count; CVA, cerebral vascular accident; CXR, chest x-ray; ECG, electrocardiogram; ECT, electroconvulsive therapy; Hb, hemoglobin; Hct, hematocrit; PT, prothrombin time; PTT, partial thromboplastin time

---

[7] What the paper calls cancellations are really delays. No surgery was fully cancelled.
[8] 2/4 admitted sexual activity prior to test; 1/4 admitted to the possibility of being pregnant prior to test

Table C-21. Noncomparative studies: Procedure or anesthesia delay

Author, Year, PMID	Study Design	Outcome Definition	Arm	N Analyzed	Counts (%)
Population: Adults					
Surgery: Cataract					
Test: Combined Panel					
Phillips, 2013 23508220	Prospective cohort	Surgical delay	Routine	530	19 (4%)
Surgery: General/Various					
Test: Biochemical Panel					
Perez 1995 7718366	Retrospective cohort	Delay operation	Routine	2784	5 (0.2%)
Test: Cardiac Stress Test					
Carliner 1986 3719447	Prospective cohort	Surgery postponed because of markedly positive exercise tests and therefore excluded from further analysis	Per Protocol	200	1 (1.0%)
Test: CXR					
Bhuripanyo 1990 2345323	Retrospective cohort	NR	Routine	933	19 (2.0%)
Test: ECG					
Correll 2009 19417620	Retrospective cohort	Postponement since ECG could not be performed and read prior to case	Per Protocol	284	3 (1.1%)
Test: Hemostasis Tests					
Perez 1995 7718366	Retrospective cohort	Delay operation	Routine (Test: PT, PTT, CBC)	3089	3 (0.1%)
Aghajanian 1991 1923209	Retrospective cohort	Implied: "changes in perioperative management"	Routine (Test: PT)	1546	0 (0%)
Test: Panel					
Golub 1992 1595835	Retrospective cohort	NR / Not unnecessary delay / Proved to be unnecessary delays due to abnormal test results that affected neither patient management nor outcome.	Routine	325 / 325 / 325	5 (1.5%)[9] / 1 (0.3%)[10] / 4 (1.2%)[11]
Kaplan 1985 3999339	Retrospective cohort	Implied by "alterations in patient care"	Routine	610	0 (0%)
Johnson 2002 12190758	Prospective cohort	Implied	Routine	100	0 (0%)

[9] Not including 2 delays due to ad hoc ECGs; however the tests that resulted in the unnecessary delay in 4 were not reported
[10] Newly diagnosed diabetes mellitus
[11] May include delays due to ad hoc tests

Author, Year, PMID	Study Design	Outcome Definition	Arm	N Analyzed	Counts (%)
Alsumait 2002 12116695	Prospective cohort	"Surgical delays"	Routine	137	0 (0%)
Narr 1991 1899710	Retrospective cohort	NR	Routine	3782	0 (0%)
Test: Pregnancy Test					
Kahn 2008 18349183	Retrospective cohort	Cancelled on day of surgery but completed at a later date	Routine	2593	5 (0.2%)
Surgery: Head & Neck/ ENT					
Test: Panel					
Haug 1999 9915390	Prospective cohort	NR	Routine	380	2 (0.5%)[12]
Surgery: Neurosurgery					
Test: Panel					
Mantha 2005 15721730	Prospective cohort	Outcome implied only (based on other related outcomes being reported)	Routine	127[13]	0 (0%)
Surgery: Orthopedic					
Test: Hemostasis Tests					
Bushick 1989 2585157	Retrospective cohort	NR	Routine	640	1 (0.2%)[14]
Test: Urinalysis					
Lawrence 1988 3377621	Retrospective cohort	NR	Routine	200	1 (0.5%)[15]
Surgery: Vascular					
Test: Cardiac Stress Test					
Van Damme 1997 9158124	Prospective cohort	Procedure postponed and myocardial revascularization was performed.	Routine	150	5 (3.3%)
Test: CXR					
Tape 1988 3339483	Retrospective cohort	Surgical delay related to CXR	Routine	341	4 (1.2%)[16]
Population: Pediatrics					
Surgery: General/Various					
Test: CXR					
Sane 1977 917629	Prospective cohort	NR	Routine	1500	11 (0.7%)[17]
Test: CBC					

[12] 1 positive pregnancy test, elevated glucose in patient with diabetes mellitus
[13] Of 1395 tests performed, 37% were indicated
[14] Elevated PTT yielded diagnosis of circulating lupus anticoagulant and 8 day postponement of surgery.
[15] Delay time 13 days
[16] Based on Table 4. Not including patient 9 whose surgical course was not based on a CXR misread as normal.
[17] 10/11 had surgery 1 month later after CXRs returned to normal (large pneumonic consolidations); 1 child moved and was lost to followup.

Author, Year, PMID	Study Design	Outcome Definition	Arm	N Analyzed	Counts (%)
Roy 1991 1714052	Retrospective cohort	Case deferred	Routine (Test: Hb)	2000	3 (0.2%)[18]
O'Connor 1990 2301750	Retrospective cohort	NR	Routine (Test: Hb/MCV)	484	2 (0.4%)[19]
			Routine (Test: WBC)	484	0 (0%)
Test: Pregnancy Test					
Malviya 1996 8831334	Prospective cohort	Surgical procedure delayed while awaiting pregnancy test results	Routine	444	10 (2.3%)
		Delay, with subsequent negative pregnancy test	Routine	444	10 (2.3%)
Azzam 1996 8712424	Retrospective cohort	NR	Routine	207	0 (0%)
Test: Urinalysis					
O'Connor 1990 2301750	Retrospective cohort	NR	Routine	453	2 (0.4%)[20]
Surgery: Head & Neck/ ENT					
Test: CBC					
Hoare 1993 8289005	Cohort (unclear)	Procedure postponed for between 2-3 months and given oral iron therapy	Routine (Test: Hb)	372	10 (2.7%)
Surgery: Orthopedic					
Test: Panel					
Ipp 2011 21926874	Retrospective cohort	Delayed until they underwent surgery to repair their cardiac lesion.	Routine	212	2 (0.9%)

Abbreviations: CABG, coronary artery bypass grafting; CBC, complete blood count; CXR, chest x-ray; ECG, electrocardiogram; Hb, hemoglobin; Hct, hematocrit; MCV, mean corpuscular volume; NR, not reported; PT, prothrombin time; PTT, partial thromboplastin time; UIT, urinary tract infection; WBC, white blood cell count

---

[18] Subgroups analysis shows that all 3 events occurred in those patients 1-5 years old.
[19] 2- and 21-months-old, delayed by 1 and 2 months, following iron therapy.
[20] 2 3-month-olds, both treated for UTIs: 1 postponed but required emergency surgery 1 week later; 1 delayed 2 months.

Table C-22. Noncomparative studies: Change in patient management

Author, Year, PMID	Study Design	Outcome Definition	Arm	N Analyzed	Counts (%)
Population: Adults					
Surgery:					
General/Various					
Test: CBC					
Bhuripanyo 1995 7622976	Prospective cohort	NR	Routine	384	38 (9.9%)
Test: CXR					
Bhuripanyo 1990 2345323	Retrospective cohort	Medical consultation, additional investigation or treatment because of the abnormality found, and the anesthesiologist decision to change treatment plan [kept because of subgroup analyses]	Routine	933	74 (7.9%)
Silvestri 1999 10713868	Prospective cohort	Deemed "useful" by anesthesiologist and leading to change in anesthetic management (72%) or to "further evaluation" (26%) or a not available reason (2%) [included because of subgroup analyses]	Per Protocol	5893	298 (5.1%)
Test: ECG					
Bhuripanyo 1992 1293256	Prospective cohort	Medical consultation, drugs administrated, postponement or cancellation, changes in the anesthetic method or medication (only outcome; with subgroup analysis)	Routine	395	10 (2.5%)

Abbreviations: CBC, complete blood count; CXR, chest x-ray; ECG, electrocardiogram; NR, not reported

Table C-23. Noncomparative studies: Change in surgical technique

Author, Year, PMID	Study Design	Outcome Definition	Arm	N Analyzed	Counts (%)
Population: Adults					
Surgery:					
General/Various					
Test: Panel					
Charpak 1988 3339918	Prospective cohort	Surgery was modified	Per Protocol	3866	1 (0.03%)
Perez 1995 7718366	Retrospective cohort	Change to surgical technique	Routine	2784	0 (0%)
Test: Hemostasis Tests					
Perez 1995 7718366	Retrospective cohort	Change to surgical technique	Routine (Test: PT, PTT, CBC)	3089	0 (0%)
Surgery: Vascular					
Test: Cardiac Stress Test					
Van Damme 1997 9158124	Prospective cohort	Planned surgery changed to another procedure	Routine	150	1 (0.7%)[21]
Population: Pediatrics					
Surgery:					
General/Various					
Test: CXR					
Sane 1977 917629	Prospective cohort	NR	Routine	1500	0 (0%)

Abbreviations: CBC, complete blood count; CXR, chest x-ray; NR, not reported; PT, prothrombin time; PTT, partial thromboplastin time

---

[21] Planned aortoiliac bypass changed to an extra-anatomic bypass graft

Table C-24. Noncomparative studies: Duration of surgical delay

Author, Year, PMID	Study Design	Outcome Definition	Arm	N Analyzed	Mean [Median] (95% CI), weeks
Population: Pediatrics					
Surgery: Head & Neck / ENT					
Test: CBC					
Hoare 1993 8289005	Cohort (unclear)	Excluding 2 patients who ultimately had surgery cancelled	Routine (Test: Hb)	8	10.6 [12] (7-13)

Abbreviations: CBC, complete blood count; Hb, hemoglobin; Hct, hematocrit

Appendix D. Risk of Bias

Table D-1. Randomized controlled trials: Risk of bias

Study Author Year PMID	Overall Risk of Bias	Elig Crit	Inapp Excl	Highly Select	Pt Charact	Outcomes	Blinding	Dropout	ITT	Multi	Discrep	Random'n	Alloc Conc	Spec Out
Cavallini 2004 15506597	Low	Yes	Yes	No	No	Yes	nd	Yes	Yes	NA	Yes	Yes	Yes	No
Chung 2009 19151274	Low	Yes	Yes	No	Yes	No	Yes	Yes	Yes	NA	Yes	Yes	nd	No
Falcone 2003 14689407	Low	Yes	Yes	No	Yes	Yes	Yes	Yes	Yes	NA	Yes	Yes	No	No
Leonard 1975 1095116	Medium	Yes	Yes	No	No	Yes	Yes	Yes	nd	NA	Yes	nd	nd	No
Lira 2001 11558245	Low	Yes	Yes	No	Yes	Yes	Yes	Yes	Yes	NA	Yes	nd	nd	No
Schein 2000 10639549	Medium	Yes	Yes	No	Yes	Yes	nd	Yes	Yes	No	Yes	nd	nd	No

Elig Crit: Eligibility criteria—Were eligibility criteria clear?
Inapp Excl: Inappropriate Exclusions—Did the study avoid inappropriate exclusions?
Highly Select: Highly Selective—Was this a highly selected, non-representative cohort of patients?
Pt Charact: Patient Characteristics—Adequate of description of patient characteristics?
Outcomes Def: Outcomes Defined—Were all the outcomes fully defined?
Blinding: Outcome Assessor Blinding—Blinded outcome assessment?
Dropout: Dropout—Dropout rate <20%?
ITT: Intention to Treat—Was there an intention to treat analysis?
Multi: Multicenter—If multicenter, was this accounted for in the analysis?
Discrep: Clearness of Reporting—Clear reporting with no discrepancies?
Random'n: Randomization—Was there an appropriate randomization technique?
Alloc Conc: Allocation Concealment—Was there allocation concealment?
Spec Out: Specific Outcome Downgrading—Should any specific outcome be further downgraded for quality issues specific to that outcome? If so, describe which and why in the comment box.
Abbreviations: nd=not documented

Table D-2. Nonrandomized comparative studies: Risk of bias

Study Author Year PMID	Overall Risk of Bias	Elig Crit	Inapp Excl	Highly Select	Pt Charact	Outcomes	Blinding	Dropout	Multi	Discrep	Nonexp Cohort	Adjust
Almanaseer 2005 15528897	High	Yes	Yes	No	Yes	Yes	nd	Yes	NA	Yes	Yes	No
Finegan 2005 15983141	High	Yes	Yes	No	No	No	Yes	Yes	NA	No	Yes	No
Larocque 1994	High	Yes	Yes	No	Yes	No	No	Yes	NA	Yes	Yes	No
Mancuso 1999 10203622	High	Yes	Unclear	No	Yes	Yes	nd	Unsure	NA	Yes	Yes	No
Meneghini 1998 9483592	High	Yes	Yes	No	No	Yes	No	Yes	NA	Yes	Yes	No
Mignonsin 1996 8762245	High	No	Unclear	No	Yes	Yes	No	Yes	NA	Yes	Yes	No
Wyatt 1989 2729769	High	Yes	Yes	No	No	Yes	nd	Yes	NA	Yes	Yes	No
Zwack 1997 9051441	High	No	Unclear	Unsure	No	Yes	nd	Yes	NA	Yes	Yes	No

Elig Crit: Eligibility criteria—Were eligibility criteria clear?
Inapp Excl: Inappropriate Exclusions—Did the study avoid inappropriate exclusions?
Highly Select: Highly Selective—Was this a highly selected, non-representative cohort of patients?
Pt Charact: Patient Characteristics—Adequate of description of patient characteristics?
Outcomes Def: Outcomes Defined—Were all the outcomes fully defined?
Blinding: Outcome Assessor Blinding—Blinded outcome assessment?
Dropout: Dropout—Dropout rate <20%?
Multi: Multicenter: If multicenter, was this accounted for in the analysis?
Discrep: Clearness of Reporting–Clear reporting with no discrepancies?
Nonexp Coh: Nonexposed Cohort Selection: Was the nonexposed cohort drawn from the same community as the exposed cohort?
Adjust: Adjustments–Was the analysis adjusted for baseline characteristics?
nd=not documented